M. A. de Kock

# DYNAMIC BRONCHOSCOPY

With a Foreword by W. T. Ulmer

With 197 Illustrations,
Most in Color

Springer-Verlag
Berlin Heidelberg New York 1977

Machiel Adriaan de Kock
M.B., Ch.B., M.Med., F.C.P. (S.A.), F.R.C.P., M.D., F.A.C.C.P.

Professor and Head of the Department of Medicine and the Respiratory Unit. University of Stellenbosch Medical School and Tygerberg Hospital

Director of the Diffuse Obstructive Pulmonary. Disease Research Group of the South African Medical Research Council
Tygerberg, South Africa

ISBN 3-540-08109-7 Springer-Verlag Berlin Heidelberg New York
ISBN 0-387-08109-7 Springer-Verlag New York Heidelberg Berlin

Library of Congress Cataloging in Publication Data. De Kock, Machiel Adriaan, 1927–. Dynamic bronchoscopy. Includes index. 1. Bronchoscope and bronchoscopy. I. Title. RC734.B7D45 616.2′3′0754 77-7906



Reproduction of the figures: Gustav Dreher GmbH, Stuttgart.

Typesetting, printing, and bookbinding by Universitätsdruckerei H. Stürtz AG, Würzburg
2121/3130-543210

# *Foreword*

Bronchoscopy means pictures: but to comprehend an image we have to learn to see. These excellent photographs, all taken by the author himself, not only instruct us in the art of seeing just about all there is to see in the bronchial system but also illustrate many relationships between visual appearances and the clinical situation. They go even further in correlating bronchoscopic findings with the function of the lung. Treated in this way, the image comes alive.

Anyone who has come to know DE KOCK as a brilliant clinician, or who has worked with him in the lung function laboratory—he has made important contributions in this field also—would have expected him to produce a monograph of this calibre. Now we have such a book.

It contains the selected results of many years' solid work. Due attention is, of course, also accorded the merits of the various bronchoscopic techniques which provide the essential background to satisfactory results.

In writing this book DE KOCK has succeeded in projecting a vivid image of the bronchi and the functional lung into our mind's eye. This work undoubtedly opens new prospects in improved care of our patients.

Bochum, Federal Republic of Germany  W.T. ULMER
Summer 1977

# *Acknowledgements*

It is the ability to take photographs through the bronchoscope which has made this book possible. The author is therefore truly grateful to the late Mr. H. Nel of Keetmanshoop, South-West Africa, for making funds available for the acquisition of the light source, optical telescopes, and photographic equipment at a time when hospital administrators could not appreciate the benefits to be derived from photography of the airways.

A major part of the work on the subject of collapsing airways was carried out with the support of the South African Medical Research Council (S.A.M.R.C.). The author is especially grateful to the President of the S.A.M.R.C., Prof. A.J. Brink, whose encouragement and support led to the establishment of the Diffuse Obstructive Pulmonary Syndrome Research Group under the Council's auspices.

Technical developments are often taken for granted, but the author is grateful to Mr. Storz of the Karl Storz KG, Tuttlingen, West Germany for his help in establishing certain techniques and for effecting necessary modifications to instruments. It is also true that any set of instruments, however well designed, often requires further modification to suit local conditions and preferences. For help in this respect the author will always be indebted to Mr. J. Ellis, Chief Technician of the Lung Unit of the Tygerberg Hospital.

The mounting and filing of a large number of photographs necessarily occupies a considerable amount of time. For undertaking this work, Miss I. Fourie of the Lung Unit has earned my thanks.

A book of this kind would be much less effective without illustrative line drawings, and in this regard I am most grateful to Cynthia E. du Plooy of the Medical Illustration Service of the Department of Didactics of the University of Stellenbosch Medical School, not only for making the drawings but also for offering her expert advice.

I am grateful to my secretary, Mrs. E. Kritzinger, for patiently retyping the manuscript many times on account of innumerable revisions of the text. I am personally indebted to Dr. C.M. Lewis for reading the text and for his constructive criticisms.

Inevitably, when one embarks on a project of this kind, the extra time required is taken from the time spent with one's family. I am therefore most grateful to my family for their understanding and encouragement.

Tygerberg, South Africa
Summer 1977

M.A. de Kock

*Contents*

# *Dynamic Bronchoscopy*

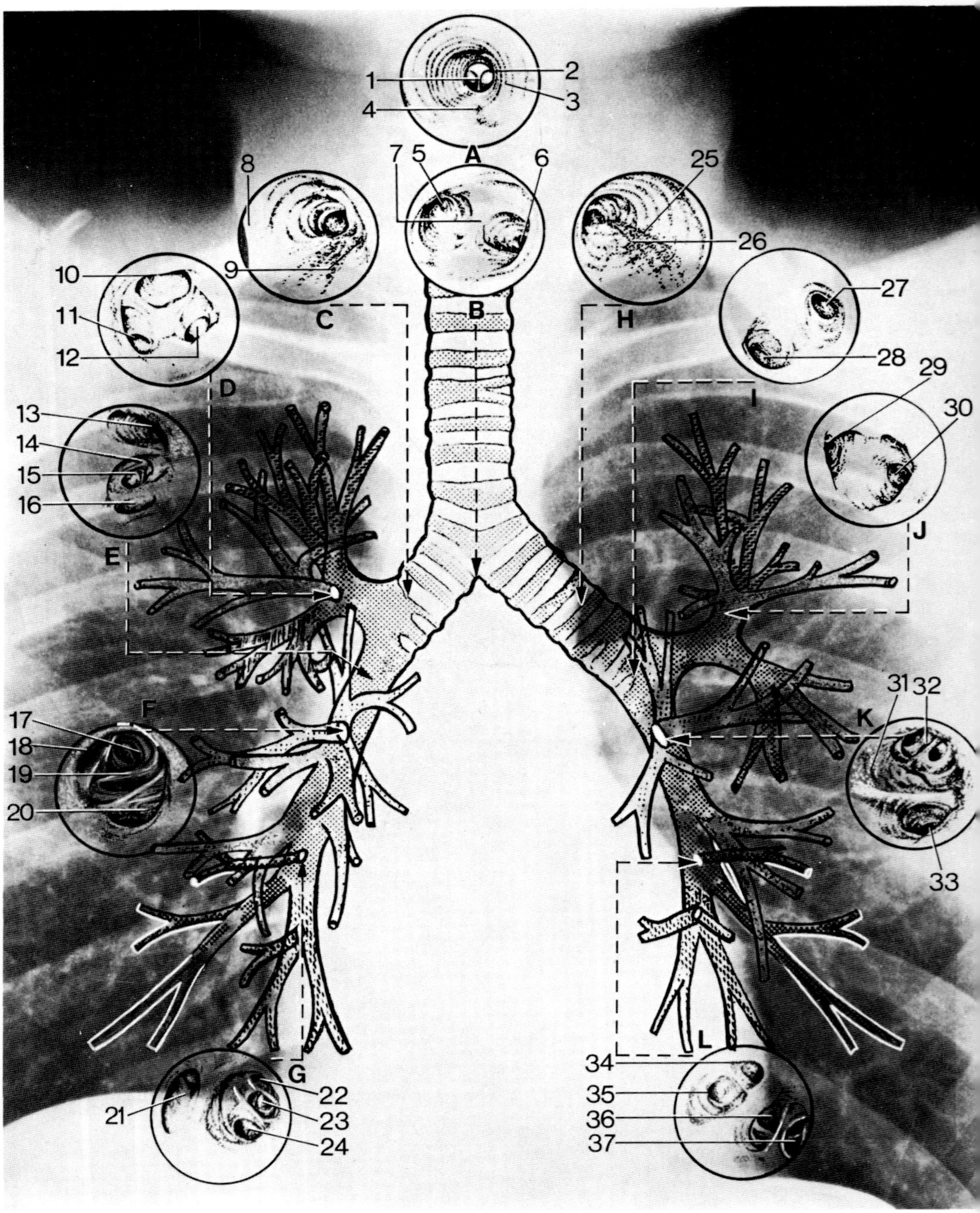

A
B
C
D
E
F
G
H
I
J
K
L
1
2
3
4
5
6
7
8
9
10
11
12
13
14
15
16
17
18
19
20
21
22
23
24
25
26
27
28
29
30
31
32
33
34
35
36
37

# Introduction

The indications for a diagnostic investigation in medicine are to some extent determined by the ease of its performance. More important, however, are the risk to the patient and the degree of discomfort inherent in the procedure. It is moreover also true that increasing operator proficiency and experience will enhance the value of the information gained and widen the scope of, and indications for, the procedure. While the technique of bronchoscopy may well be slightly more difficult than, for instance, that of sigmoidoscopy, the reluctance of many physicians concerned with chest disease to make greater use of the bronchoscope to aid the more complete assessment of patients with respiratory complaints is somewhat incomprehensible. Although the removal of foreign bodies from the bronchial tree and the diagnosis of intrabronchial tumors remain prime indications for bronchoscopy, they certainly are not the sole indications. Employing local anesthesia and more sophisticated modern anesthetic methods, the investigator can examine patients during normal respiration and make a detailed study of func-

---

◁ *A. Trachea*

1. Left main bronchus
2. Right main bronchus
3. Cartilages
4. Membranous posterior wall

*B. Trachea at level of carina*

5. Left main bronchus
6. Right main bronchus
7. Carina

*C. Right main bronchus at level of carina*

8. Carina
9. Opening to right upper lobe bronchus

*D. Opening to right upper lobe bronchus*

10. Anterior segmental bronchus
11. Posterolateral segmental bronchus
12. Apical segmental bronchus

*E. Right intermediate bronchus*

13. Middle lobe bronchus
14. 15. Basal bronchi
16. Apical segmental bronchus of lower lobe

*F. Right lower lobe bronchus*

17. Basal bronchi
18. Medial basal segmental bronchus
19. Subapical segmental bronchus
20. Apical lower segmental bronchus

*G. Basal segments of right lower lobe*

21. Medial basal segmental bronchus
22. Anterior basal segmental bronchus
23. Lateral basal segmental bronchus
24. Posterior basal segmental bronchus

*H. Left main bronchus at level of carina*

25. Longitudinal elastic bundles
26. Transverse muscle bundles

*I. Left main bronchus at level of left upper lobe opening*

27. Lower lobe opening
28. Upper lobe opening

*J. Left upper lobe bronchus*

29. Upper division segmental bronchus
30. Lingular segmental bronchus

*K. Left lower lobe bronchus*

31. Spur of left upper lobe bronchus
32. Basal bronchi
33. Apical segmental lower lobe bronchus

*L. Common variant of left lower lobe*

34. Medial basal segmental bronchus
35. Anterior basal segmental bronchus
36. Lateral basal segmental bronchus
37. Posterior basal segmental bronchus

tional changes. Technical developments, such as the "cold" light source and the extremely effective telescopes with their various angles of vision, have improved the rigid bronchoscope almost to perfection. The introduction and further development of the fiberoptic bronchoscope, while in no way implying redundancy of the rigid instrument, have undoubtedly extended the usefulness of bronchoscopy.

Bronchoscopy is today a well-established clinical investigation. It has received much attention in the literature and has been the subject of a number of excellent monographs published recently [1, 2]. This book has been written neither in a spirit of "me-tooism" nor in an attempt to improve on existing works on the subject of bronchoscopy. It should be viewed as an account of the personal experience gained by a clinician with a special interest in the mechanics of physiological function through bronchoscopic studies conducted over a period of 22 years. The author believes that the bronchoscope is a useful research tool which can contribute significantly to a better understanding of many pulmonary diseases. It is not merely an instrument to diagnose tumors or to remove foreign bodies from the bronchial tree.

While this book affords descriptions of the technique of bronchoscopy and of the endoscopic appearances of morbid anatomy, e.g., intrabronchial tumors, the emphasis is rather on observations of functional change and other aspects of pathology, such as trauma of the airways. Thus, the various techniques governing specific maneuvers are not detailed, and where the author does elaborate on technique, it is to explain methods personally employed without claiming originality. Although the removal of foreign bodies is an important aspect of bronchoscopy, it is a subject on its own and best learned by practical demonstration. It will therefore not be covered here. This work, furthermore, should not be viewed as a complete atlas of normal variations in bronchoscopic appearances and of bronchial pathology. The most common presentations are described, and, if these are understood, the reader should have no difficulty in recognizing and comprehending both variations of normal and different patterns of pathology.

# *Chapter 1*
# Indications for and Contraindications to Bronchoscopy

## Indications

The most generally accepted indications for bronchoscopy still remain the removal of foreign bodies from the airway and the diagnosis of intrabronchial tumors. Bronchoscopy is the single most important special investigation in establishing the diagnosis of bronchogenic carcinoma and should be performed in any patient with symptoms and signs which may be associated with malignancy of the lungs, in the absence of other diagnostic evidence, such as positive histology of samples obtained through the biopsy of lymph nodes, pleura, or other tissues.

The most suggestive presenting symptoms and signs are hemoptysis, unexplained cough, the unprovoked onset of hoarseness, the unexplained development of clubbing of the fingers, pleural effusion in patients over 40 years of age, recurrent chest infections in previously healthy patients over 40, and radiographic findings including hilar shadows, coin lesions, and atelectasis. In cases of bronchial carcinoma, bronchoscopy is indicated not only to establish or confirm the diagnosis but also to assess operability. Even in patients with patently inoperable carcinoma, the determination of histologic type is of more than academic interest: Analysis of biopsy material obtained through bronchoscopy may indicate prognosis and influence decisions on palliation by radiotherapy and/or chemotherapy.

Important indications for bronchoscopy, other than those relating to foreign bodies and suspected tumors are:

1. Postoperative segmental or lobar collapse.
2. The aftermath of severe chest trauma: to exclude lacerations and to clear the airways of blood clot and inhaled material prior to the institution of intermittent positive pressure respiration.
3. A history of aspiration of gastric contents.
4. Prolonged coma, where it may be important to clear the patient's airways.
5. Obstructive airways disease. Here, as will be discussed later, bronchoscopy may be of great value in the assessment of disordered structure and function.
6. Under certain conditions, e.g., following trauma to the upper airways and obstruction of the larynx, it may be technically easier to pass a bronchoscope than an intralaryngeal tube.

## Contraindications

When performed with due care by a skilled operator, bronchoscopy is seldom if ever absolutely contraindicated. Dislocation of the neck or fractures of cervical vertebrae and recent myocardial infarction should, however, be regarded in this light. It is the author's firm belief that general anesthesia, with the consequent suppression of respiration, should not be employed in the investigation of the critically ill or poor-risk patient. Local anesthesia and/or intravenously administered diazepam provide a safe and usually adequate alternative in such cases. The rigid bronchoscope, moreover, offers the critically ill patient an "open" airway, and additionally provides, through an inlet port, a free-flowing supply of oxygen for the duration of the procedure. Both factors are especially advantageous in such patients. Relative contraindications to bronchoscopy exist in respect to the elderly, extremely ill, or intensely dyspnoeic patient, these being determined, as is the case with all invasive investigations, by weighing the specific risk factors against the need to obtain diagnostic information. For instance, bronchoscopic investigation with a view to the histological typing of lung carcinoma radiologically assessed as totally inoperable, is probably not justifiable in these circumstances; whereas, the need to aspirate bronchial secretions in order to relieve distress may well outweigh negative considerations in patients of this kind. Bronchoscopy in a patient presenting features of the syndrome of superior vena caval obstruction should be approached with great caution and should indeed be avoided wherever possible. Edema of the glottis or uncontrolled hemorrhage, or both, are very real complications. A 4.5-mm fiberoptic bronchoscope is probably safer than a rigid instrument under these circumstances.

# *Chapter 2* Equipment and Technique

While bronchoscopy can, under emergency conditions, be performed in the patient's bed in a general ward, accurate diagnosis demands an adequately equipped room set aside for this specific purpose (Fig. I). It is hardly necessary to stress that, in addition to the requisite anesthetic equipment, full essential resuscitative instrumentation should be available. Although not indispensable, cardiac monitoring equipment is useful, as are facilities for arterial blood-gas analysis where required. The availability of radiographic screening facilities, ideally an image-intensifier mounted on a C-shaped arm which encircles the patient and closed-circuit television monitoring linked to a 70-mm camera, widens the scope of bronchoscopy and improves diagnostic accuracy. These facilities make selective bronchography possible when required, and catheters and brushes or the fiberoptic bronchoscope can be guided into specific lung segments with greater ease.

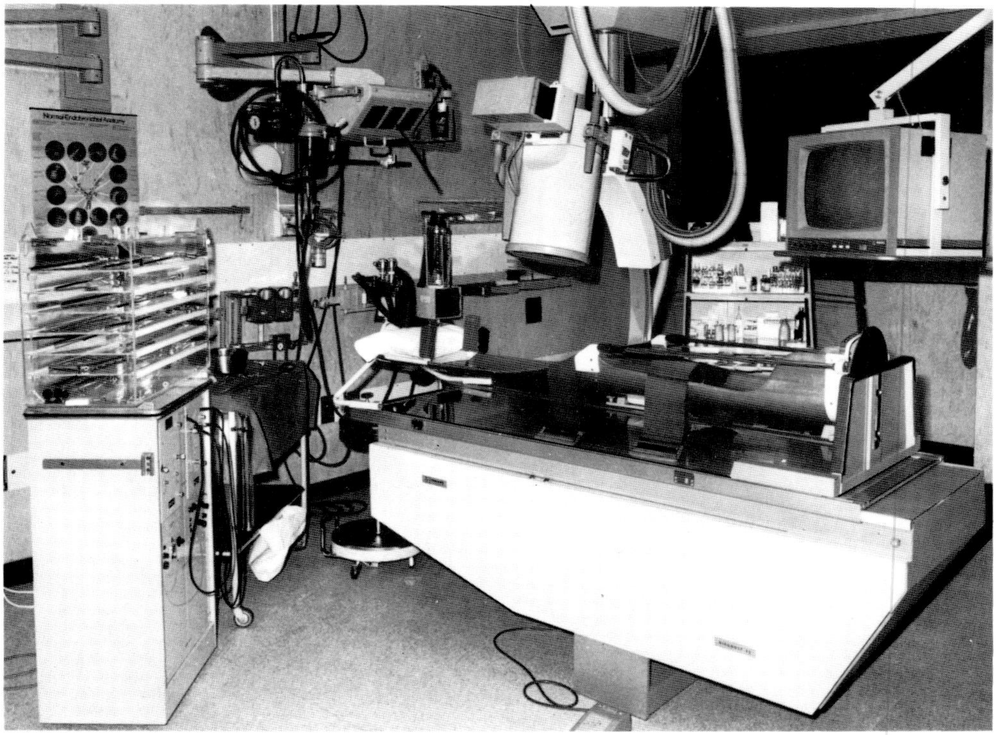

Fig. I. Bronchoscopy theater with screening equipment

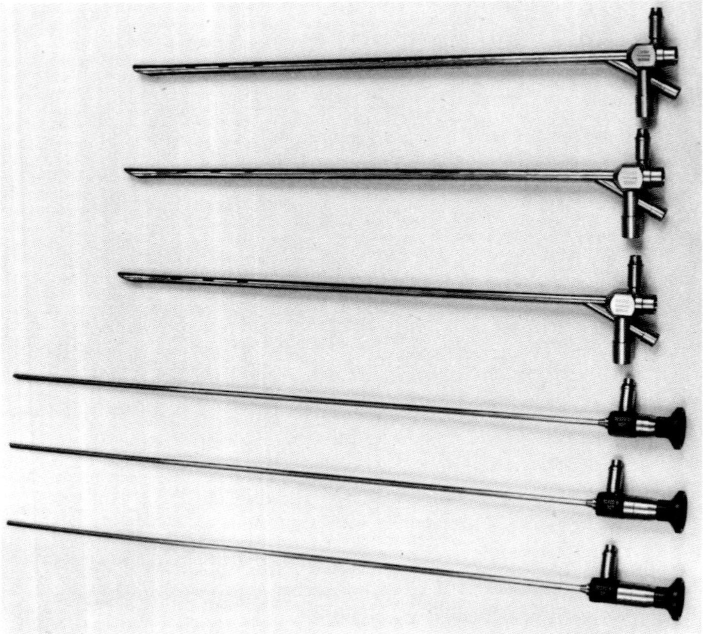

Fig. II. Bronchoscopes of 8.5 mm, 7.5 mm, and 6.5 mm caliber for adult use, with matching freely interchangeable 90°-, 30°-, and 0°-angled viewing telescopes

a

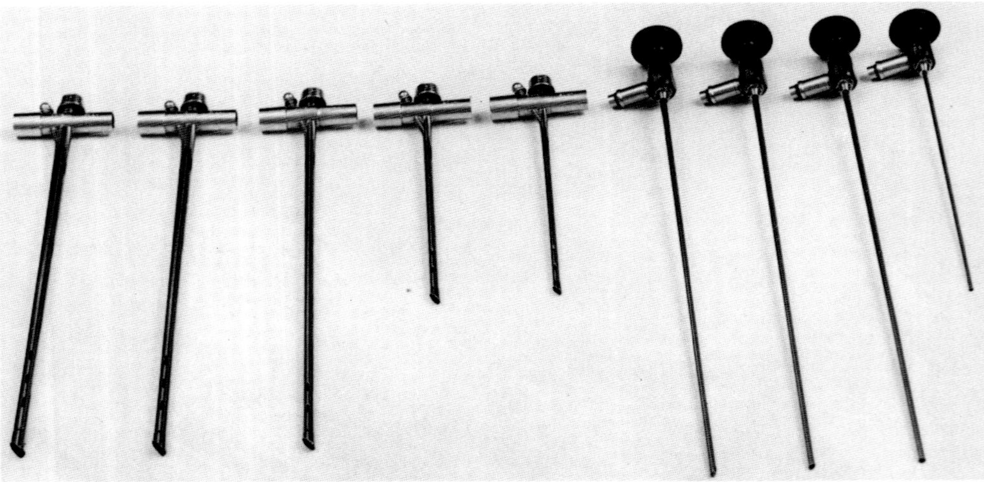

b

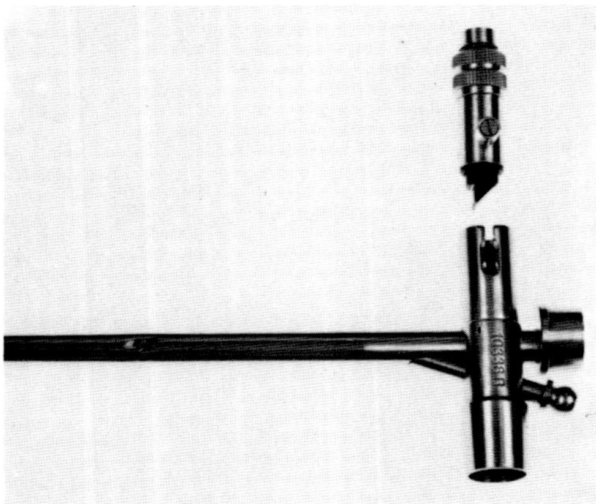

Fig. III. (a) Bronchoscopes of 6 mm, 5 mm, 4 mm, 3.5 mm, and 3 mm caliber for use in younger children and infants, with telescopes 30 cm in length and having angles of vision of 0°, 30°, and 70° for use with the larger three sizes, and a 20-cm forward-viewing (0°) telescope for use with the smaller caliber bronchoscopes. (b) The prismatic attachment to the light source, which projects light down the shaft of the bronchoscope in pediatric usage

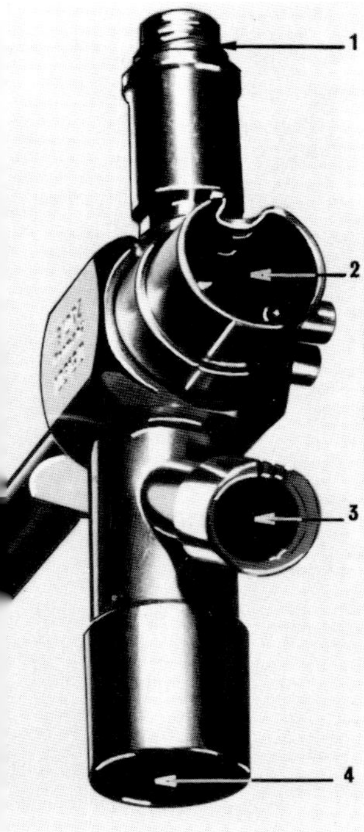


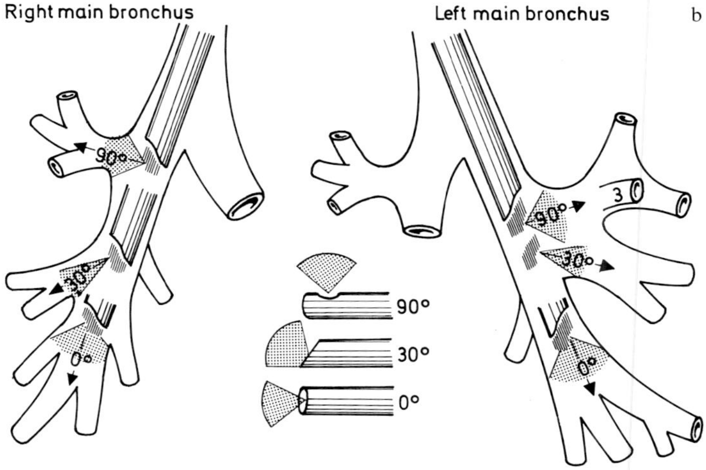


Fig. IV. (a) Operator's end of Storz bronchoscope. *1* Adaptor for cold light source; *2* observer port; *3* Inlet for passing catheters. The Sanders Venturi injector can be applied here; *4* inlet port for the administration of oxygen or anesthetic gases. (b) Telescopes with 0°, 30°, and 90° angles of vision are necessary for a complete bronchoscopic examination. Vision to at least the level of the segmental and the first subsegmental bronchi is possible

The development of the cold-light system as adapted to the rigid bronchoscope represented a major advance in technology. Where a theater is to be equipped for the purpose of bronchoscopic examinations, the capital expenditure on the best available light source is amply justified. A system which incorporates the facility of switching to a reserve light bulb in the event of failure of the bulb in use, will avert irksome delays and inconvenience.

Rigid bronchoscopes are available in many different calibers. The 8.5-mm and 7.5-mm sizes are suitable for most adults and adolescents (Fig. II). In general, the largest bronchoscope which can be passed with ease through the vocal chords should be used. Smaller sizes ranging in caliber from 6 mm through 5 mm, 4 mm, 3.5 mm to 3 mm are obtainable for use in younger children and infants (Fig. III a). The light source of these smaller bronchoscopes derives from prismatic projection from the handle down the shaft of the instrument (Fig. III b).

The bronchoscope should incorporate a separate inlet port for the administration of oxygen or anesthetic gases and a smaller channel through which catheters can be passed (Fig. IV a). All bronchoscopes have beveled tips, with the longer lip positioned on the same side as the handle of the instrument. For complete flexibility in technique, the operator should have at his disposal telescopes with at least the 0°, 30°, and 90° angles of vision (Fig. IV b) in all necessary sizes.

The fiberoptic bronchoscope contributes to the effectiveness of the endoscopic procedure, and with the smaller caliber flexible instruments (4.5 mm and 3.5 mm), a large proportion of more peripherally sited tumors can be visualized. Arguments concerning the exclusive employment of either the rigid bronchoscope or the fiberoptic instrument are irrelevant and illogical. The two instruments are definitely complementary, and each is essential in its own right. For most routine work the rigid bronchoscope is preferred, and with the available telescopes, endoscopic vision up to at least segmental level is entirely adequate. Biopsy samples may be obtained from the lobar bronchi and even from the primary segmental bronchi by means of a specially designed forceps. Manipulation through distorted airways and the entry of subsegmental bronchi underline the design characteristics of the fiberoptic bronchoscope. The flexible instrument is also most usefully employed in bronchoscopic examination through a tracheostomy tube or a previously positioned endotracheal tube. The indications for and the extent of the use made of the two types of bronchoscopes will naturally reflect the individual preferences of the operator. Many experienced bronchoscopists have the best of both worlds by embarking on a study with the rigid bronchoscope and subsequently passing the selective fiberoptic modality through the rigid instrument to inspect the segmental bronchi as desired.

## Anesthesia

It may be claimed that the risks to the patient posed by bronchoscopy are, where they exist, related rather to the anesthetic employed than to the bronchoscopic manipulation itself. Local anesthesia is undoubtedly safer than general anesthesia, although the latter is much more comfortable for the patient. The use of modern techniques, for example the Venturi injection technique of Sanders (Sanders, 1967; Stradling, 1973), renders even general anesthesia with muscle relaxation relatively safe. It is advantageous to have the patient breathing spontaneously, not only from the point of view of safety, but also because the observation of functional changes during respiration is possible. This is the most cogent reason for preferring the combination of local anesthesia and intravenous diazepam and/or neurolept anesthesia in most instances.

Where bronchoscopy is indicated in the seriously ill or comatose patient in order to remove excess secretions, minimal anesthesia is desirable, and intravenous diazepam is probably the safest form.

The role of atropine in bronchoscopy is somewhat controversial. While its prophylactic use to counteract the vagal stimulation produced by manipulations in the upper airway would seem desirable, negative aspects include its inspissating effect on bronchial secretions and a direct physiological action on the bronchi capable of obscuring preexisting and reflex-reactive functional changes. In order to minimize these undesirable effects, atropine should therefore preferably be administered by intravenous injection of 0.4–0.6 mg immediately prior to the commencement of the procedure, and not in the form of a premedication.

While the specific anesthetic technique employed depends on the experience and preference of the anesthetist and the condition of the patient and extent of the procedure planned, the methods discussed below have proved satisfactory and extremely safe.

### Local Anesthesia and Intravenous Diazepam

The tongue, the soft palate, the oropharynx, and the vocal chords are sprayed with a 4% lignocaine (lidocaine, xylocaine) solution, utilizing a laryngoscope to gain access to the epiglottis and the glottis. As soon as local anesthesia has been accomplished, diazepam in a dosage of 0.4 mg/kg (optimum total in the range of 20–30 mg) is administered by rapid intravenous injection, the patient having been forewarned of a likely burning sensation in the arm above the injection site. It is, however, important to individualize the dose of diazepam in terms of the patient's age and cardiorespiratory status, and its hypnotic effect may be titrated against the development of ptosis on upward glance and the abolition of the eyelash reflex, both usually reliable signs of adequate anesthesia. While the patient may still react to stimuli and may cough, he should experience total amnesia in respect to the procedure. A bronchoscope may now be passed through the vocal chords into the upper part of the trachea. Slight coughing is frequently elicited, but this subsides when the bronchoscope has been held stationary for a few seconds. By means of a Clerf atomiser, the trachea is sprayed with 4% lignocaine through the bronchoscope, which is then advanced further down the trachea. The carina and subsequent bronchial branchings are more richly supplied with cough receptors, and they are thus more sensitive to mechanical stimulation. The carina and main bronchi should therefore be sprayed directly before the major bronchial passages are entered. Grossly inflamed mucous membranes are relatively insensitive to local anesthetic action, and when secretions are present in the main airways, suction should be employed to remove this coating layer prior to the application of local anesthesia. In order to avoid toxic effects consequent upon systemic absorption, the total dose of lignocaine should be limited to 500 mg or approximately 12 ml of the 4% solution.

### Local Anesthesia Plus Neurolept Anesthesia with Intravenous Diazepam Administration

When a prolonged procedure is anticipated, or where technical difficulties are likely to be encountered, perhaps in relation to patient noncooperation, the following method may prove useful.

Droperidol in a dosage of 0.1 mg/kg is administered intravenously immediately prior to the application of local anesthesia in the manner already described. This is followed, some 10 min later, by the intravenous injection of fentanyl in a dosage of 0.001 mg/kg and a rapid injection of diazepam in the 0.4-mg/kg dosage recommended above. Here, too, the anesthetic dose should be individualized, taking into account the patient's age, and in the case of fentanyl, it may be titrated against the respiratory frequency. Doses up to 0.002 mg/kg are sometimes required.

Introduction of the bronchoscope at this juncture should be followed by further local anesthetic spraying as already outlined. Droperidol may cause anxiety in some patients, and where this is observed, diazepam should be given sooner. Fentanyl should preferably not be used in elderly patients or in patients with respiratory failure. Neurolept anesthesia can be administered without the use of diazepam. KELLER and co-workers recommend the use of droperidol in a dosage of 0.15 mg/kg, to be followed 3 min later by a 0.005-mg/kg dose of fentanyl, both to be administered intravenously [4].

### Propanidid

Propanidid (Fabantol) is a very useful ultra-short-acting nonbarbituric agent for intravenous use in a dosage of 7 mg/kg. It may be employed as an adjunct to anesthesia if difficulties are encountered in passing the bronchoscope or the procedure has to be extended. Intermittent administration is recommended, governed by the length of the procedure. It has considerable analgesic properties and also exerts a hyperventilatory effect, which may prove useful during bronchography.

### Inhalational Anesthesia in Combination with Local Anesthesia

Inhalational anesthesia in combination with local anesthesia is preferred for infants and younger children, especially when foreign bodies are to be removed from the bronchial tree.

## Manipulation of the Bronchoscope

An essential prerequisite in the acquisition of bronchoscopic technique is complete familiarity with the anatomy, not only of the bronchial tree but also that of the back of the throat and the larynx. Although many experienced bronchoscopists utilize a laryngoscope to insert the bronchoscope through the vocal chords, the novice should be encouraged to master the technique of passing the bronchoscope directly. The anatomy, as viewed through the bronchoscope, and the detailed manipulative maneuvers employed will be described in the following chapter. Here it will suffice to stress a few essential points regarding the technique of manipulating the bronchoscope through the mouth and directing it distally towards the glottis and between the vocal chords. These directions should be regarded only as guidelines of a general nature, since the operator will inevitably develop individual variations as he gains experience and technical expertise.

A common tendency is to extend the head and neck too far backward. This will often result in extreme anterior displacement of the larynx, impeding vision of this structure. Optimally, the head should be positioned in extension relative to the neck, and the neck should in turn be slightly flexed on the thorax. This is most easily achieved when the head is gripped by the occiput and slightly displaced towards the thorax by means of axially exerted pressure (Fig. V).

Where the bronchoscopic examination is to be conducted under local anesthesia, the patient is requested to clear his mouth of mucus before the bronchoscope is inserted. If intravenous diazepam or general anesthesia is employed, the oral cavity should be cleared by suction of all secretions which may have accumulated at the back of the throat, and this should preferably be performed under direct vision through a laryngoscope.

The operator's left hand is the more important in controlling the movements of the patient's head and stabilizing the bronchoscope. With the middle and ring fingers of this hand crooked around the patient's upper set of teeth or gums, the weight of the bronchoscope is borne by the thumb, while the index finger is taxed with the fixation of the instrument (Fig. VI).

Care must be exercised not to exert pressure on the upper teeth or gums, and prior inspection of the teeth should be undertaken to ascertain whether there are any dental bridges or crowns which could be damaged in the course of the procedure. Both the upper and the lower lip should be retracted from the teeth or gums in order to prevent their being drawn into the mouth in the wake of the advancing bronchoscope.

The bronchoscope is manipulated by the right hand (Fig. VII) and is held with the tip of the bevel placed superiorly. Only the tip of the bronchoscope should be lubricated, and care should be exercised to avoid spilling lubricant on the end nearest the handle which would make for slippery handling, or permitting lubricant to enter the lateral ventilatory openings near the tip and obstruct vision if not removed. Manipulative movements should be deliberate but at the same time always gentle and unforced.

Fig. V. Positioning of the head by displacing the occiput towards the body with resultant extension of the head on the neck and slight flexion of the neck on the body

Fig. VI. Placement of the middle and ring fingers over the upper teeth or gums with the weight of the bronchoscope borne by the left thumb

Fig. VII. Fixation of the bronchoscope with the left hand during manipulation with the right hand

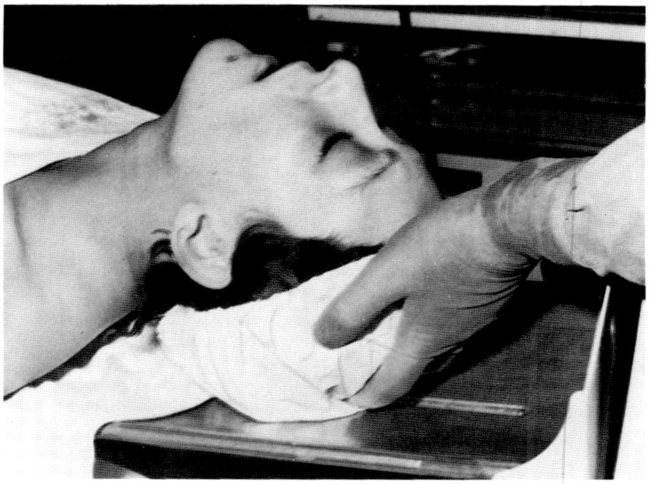

Fig. V

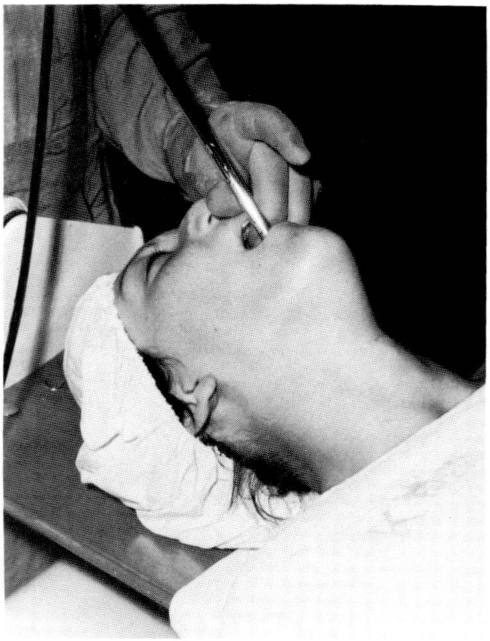

Fig. VI

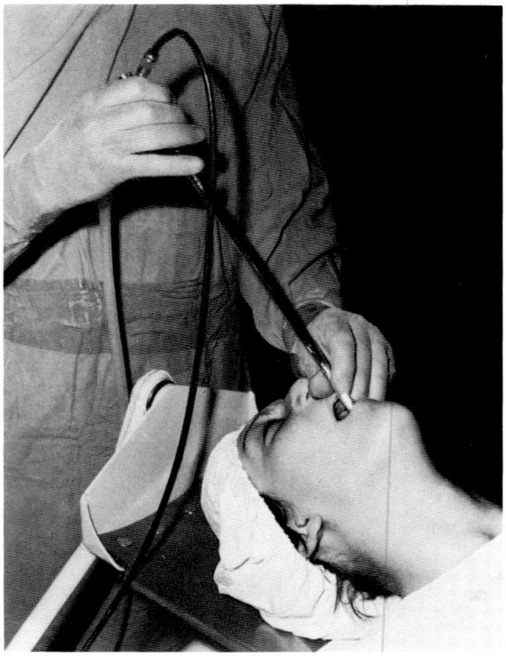

Fig. VII

The diagnostic procedure as such commences from the time the tip of the bronchoscope enters the mouth; all movements from this juncture take place under full vision from the observer's end of the bronchoscope. It is essential to maintain the midline position of the bronchoscope as it is guided over the tongue until the uvula comes into view. When local anesthesia is employed, however, it is sometimes necessary to pass the instrument to one side of the tongue to minimize mechanical stimulation, and here the tip may be centered by direct visualization of the uvula. The bronchoscope is now advanced further, the observer's end being lowered while the tip is elevated past the uvula. The epiglottis now comes into view and may be seen to rest against the posterior wall of the throat. The tip of the epiglottis is lifted by means of the distal bevel of the bronchoscope, and here the operator should take care not to advance the instrument too far in this direction, lest the glottis be missed and the bronchoscope enter the esophagus. As the tip of the epiglottis is lifted, the handle end of the bronchoscope is lowered still further until the glottis is visualized. A short epiglottis may be the cause of some difficulty, as it will tend to slip off the bevel of the bronchoscope.

It remains important to maintain a central position of the bronchoscope tip. Any difficulty encountered in visualizing the glottis can usually be ascribed to lateral displacement of the instrument's tip to the right or to the left of the pharynx or to its being advanced too far posteriorly once the epiglottis has been lifted. The bronchoscope should also not be advanced when visibility is poor, or when the operator is unable to identify the landmarks described. When the vocal chords are missed, it is advisable to withdraw the instrument and proceed from the start. Care should be exercised at all times in the avoidance of trauma and bleeding, which will not only result in discomfort to the patient at a later stage but will also complicate the procedure itself.

A step-by-step description of the normal anatomy and function of the airways as viewed through the bronchoscope in the course of a comprehensive study is provided in the ensuing chapter.

# *Chapter 3* Normal Anatomy and Function of the Airways as Seen Through the Bronchoscope

The bronchoscopic examination begins in the posterior part of the mouth and the pharynx. First the uvula is identified (Fig. 1). With the uvula as midline marker, the bronchoscope is advanced slightly anteriorly until the epiglottis can be seen (Fig. 2). When the epiglottis has been inspected, its tip is lifted anteriorly with the bevel of the bronchoscope, and the vocal chords and the larynx are then demonstrated (Fig. 3). The vocal chords are carefully inspected and their respiratory excursions observed. In the inspiratory phase the chords move apart, while in expiration they approximate.

In the course of a gag maneuver, the chords close tightly together and are covered and virtually concealed by the aryepiglottic or the vestibular folds or both, hindering recognition (Fig. 4). No attempt should be made to advance the bronchoscope through closed vocal chords (Fig. 5), as damage to these structures may ensue.

When the vocal chords draw apart in inspiration, the bronchoscope is rotated with the bevel of the instrument orientated vertically. The bevel is then inserted between the chords (Fig. 6) and firmly advanced through the opening, while the bronchoscope is rotated back to its original position. The larynx should now be inspected, and the cricoid cartilage is identified as being slightly narrower than the adjacent structures and describing a full circle (Fig. 7c). With the head and neck held in extension, the cricoid is at the level of the sixth cervical vertebra (Fig. 7a). From this point, the bronchoscope is advanced to just below the level of the cricoid cartilage. The cervical or extrathoracic trachea, which assumes near-maximum length in this extended position, may now be inspected (Fig. 8).

The cervical tracheal cartilages form the major segment of a small circle, with a narrow posterior membrane representing the minor segment of the same circle. The respiratory excursions of this posterior membrane of the cervical trachea are minimal. Normally, the cervical trachea is freely mobile, and side-to-side and anteroposterior movement is readily effected by slight pressure applied to the tip of the rigid bronchoscope. Cervical lymph nodes, enlarged by malignant infiltration, and thyroid tumors can fix the cervical trachea or distort its contour.

With the bronchoscope positioned just below the suprasternal notch at the thoracic inlet, the observer will note the progressive widening of the posterior membrane in the thoracic trachea, the widest point being reached at the level of the carina (Figs. 9 and 10). There can be considerable interindividual variation in the width of the posterior membrane at comparable levels of the thoracic trachea (Fig. 11). This may assume functional significance, since a trachea with a relatively wide posterior membrane is potentially unstable and its volume more markedly controlled by variations in intrathoracic pressure (see Chapter 4).

In the thoracic trachea the posterior membrane does indeed display movement during the respiratory cycle. In the course of inspiration the membrane is displaced

---
Figs. 1–28 see pp. 42–59

posteriorly and describes a full circle with the tracheal cartilage, while it bulges into the tracheal lumen during expiration (Fig. 12). These movements may be accentuated by deep inspiration and by forced expiratory effort such as a cough. Not only does the posterior membrane prolapse into the tracheal lumen during forced expiration, but there also occurs an inward bulging of the intercartilaginous membranes under the strain of the increased intrathoracic pressure.

It is important that the operator should observe and comprehend these movements and that he become well acquainted with the range of normal variations, since such an understanding is of great value in the assessment of pathological conditions, for instance the collapsing airways of emphysema or infiltrative disease of the airways. These dynamic events and their functional significance are described more fully in the following chapter.

The thoracic trachea shares the mobility of the cervical portion, and is capable of a similar range of movements in response to pressure applied through the tip of the rigid bronchoscope. Here too, infiltrated lymph nodes may anchor and fix the trachea.

Familiarity with the dynamic changes in the trachea is of great value when inconspicuous pathological changes are to be distinguished. Inflammatory changes, pressure exerted by enlarged, infiltrated lymph nodes, and malignant infiltration of the wall, all tend to immobilize the trachea.

## The Carina

Recognition of the carina usually presents no problem (Fig. 13). It should, however, be remembered that the right main bronchus is about one-third wider than the left and constitutes a virtual downward prolongation of the trachea, while the left main bronchus, apart from its slightly smaller caliber, differs in its acute angle of origin. It is, therefore, possible for the bronchoscope, when not advanced under continuous vision, to pass unnoticed directly into the right bronchus. This is particularly liable to occur when the left lung is partially or totally collapsed.

There is a large variation in the appearances of the normal carina, but a full range of illustrations of these differences is beyond the scope of a book of this size. The carina should, however, always be studied carefully and special attention paid to the normal respiratory excursions.

Mucosal corrugations of the posterior wall of the trachea become apparent at this level and, dividing at the carina, continue down both main bronchi, becoming more pronounced.

The carina should be sharp and knifelike. While it usually appears to be orientated vertically, it may deviate as much as 45° from the vertical. Normally, the carina widens out anteriorly and posteriorly to a fairly limited extent. It is freely mobile and can easily be displaced laterally by the tip of the rigid bronchoscope. Prior to any such manipulation, it will be recalled, the extreme sensitivity of the carina demands that it be resprayed with local anesthetic in order to forestall severe coughing.

Normally, slight movement of the carina, reflecting the transmitted pulsations of the heart, can be detected. In the course of the respiratory cycle, the carina also moves – proximally during expiration and distally during the inspiratory phase. Anteroposterior flattening of the carina is also possible during expiration (Figs. 14 and 15). The movement of the posterior tracheal membrane is usually accentuated at this level.

Inflammation may blunt the edge of the carina. Changes brought about by malignant tumors are described fully in Chapt. 5.

## Right Main Bronchus

With the beveled tip of the bronchoscope positioned just above the carina, the chin of the patient is rotated to the left, thereby displacing the tip of the bronchoscope rightward and enabling the operator to see down the right main bronchus.

The right bronchus is relatively straight, and by using the forward viewing or 0° telescope, the operator very often has a field of vision extending down to the basal bronchi (Fig. 16).

The posterior membrane of the right main bronchus is very wide, and the bronchial cartilages are almost semicircular in form. The mucosal corrugations are frequently quite pronounced. The posterior membrane here also moves into the bronchial lumen in expiration and posteriorly during inspiration. Immediately below and to the right of the carina, in the three o'clock position, lies the opening of the right upper lobe bronchus (Fig. 16). When the mucosal corrugations are prominent, those laterally disposed can frequently be seen to branch off into the upper lobe bronchial orifice (Fig. 17). If the tip of the bronchoscope or telescope is deflected slightly more laterally, the initial few millimeters of the upper lobe bronchus come into view. The spur of the opening is sharp, and during respiration it moves up and down. This movement is lacking in the presence of pathology (for instance, enlarged infiltrated lymph nodes at the origin of the upper lobe bronchus) and the bronchial spur also appears blunt and thick. When the 90°-angled telescope is employed, the upper lobe bronchus can be visualized in its entirety, and its segmental branches, namely the apical, anterior, and posterior divisions, can be identified (Fig. 18).

When the 90°-angled telescope is exchanged for the straight or 0° forward-viewing telescope, the intermediate bronchus can be visualized beyond the opening of the upper lobe bronchus (Fig. 19). The intermediate bronchus extends downwards for approximately 2 cm, at which juncture the middle lobe bronchus originates, its opening being visible in the twelve o'clock position (Fig. 20). If the 30°-angled telescope is utilized, the operator can see into the middle lobe bronchus and recognize its division into medial and lateral segments. Once again, the spur of the opening is sharp and moves on respiration. A few millimeters distal to the middle lobe bronchial origin, the opening to the apical segment of the lower lobe can be viewed in the six o'clock position (Fig. 20). The 30°-angled telescope may suffice to follow the course of the apical segment down to its subsegmental divisions, but the 90°-angled telescope is often required for this purpose. Not infrequently, a subapical segmental bronchial opening can be distinguished immediately distal to the opening to the apical lobar segment.

At this point in the course of the right bronchus, there may be an abrupt narrowing, and from here on the 7.5- or 8.5-mm bronchoscope can be advanced no further. Distal vision can, however, be extended through the use of either the 30°- or the 0°-angled telescope to embrace the four basal segmental bronchi, even to their primary subsegmental divisions (Fig. 21). All the spurs of these bronchial openings are similarly sharp and display respiratory mobility.

## Left Main Bronchus

The bronchoscope is now withdrawn to a point just above the carina and, following the rotation of the patient's head to the right, the beveled tip migrates to the left main bronchus (Fig. 22). It will be noticed immediately that the slight lateral curvature of the left bronchus precludes as extensive a distal view of this side as is possible in the right bronchus (Fig. 23).

The wide posterior membrane, analogous to that of the right bronchus, will be noted. In advancing down the left main bronchus, the bronchoscope impinges on the medial wall of the bronchus, the rigid instrument exerting a straightening effect. It is essential that no force be employed, and the bronchoscope should be advanced slowly and cautiously. Approximately 4 cm from the carina, the opening to the left upper lobe can be seen laterally in the ten o'clock position. This opening is significantly larger than that of the upper lobe bronchus on the right. On occasion this opening is partially obscured against the left wall of the bronchus, but more often it is easily seen (Fig. 24). When the 30°-angled telescope is used, it is almost invariably easy to view the course of the left upper lobe bronchus up to the openings to the lingula and the other segmental bronchi (Fig. 25).

The bronchus supplying the lingula rarely originates from a site close to the main bronchus (Fig. 26).

The apical segmental division of the left lower lobe bronchus derives from the main bronchus at a point just beyond the left upper lobe opening and is situated posteriorly at six o'clock (Fig. 27). The 90°-angled telescope is required to extend the observer's view into the segmental opening up to the subsidiary branches.

There is no discrete medial basal segmental bronchus originating from the left lower lobe bronchus. The commonest mode of divisions is into anterior, lateral, and posterior basal bronchi (Fig. 27). Many normal variations occur, the commonest of which is that the lower lobe bronchus bifurcates into two main basal branches, each of which almost immediately divides further (Fig. 28). Occasionally, it may prove extremely difficult to classify the bronchi according to any recognized distribution pattern without doing a selective bronchogram.

## Some General Comments

The above commentary affords only a brief description of the circumstances most frequently encountered. Where the bronchoscopist possesses a sound, detailed knowledge of the anatomy of the respiratory system, there will usually be no problem in the recognition of normal variations. The novice is well advised to identify by name each structure as it is encountered from the starting point of the bronchoscopy. He must pursue a steady mental commentary on the state of the mucous membrane, the presence of mucous secretions, the mobility of the trachea, the carina, and the bronchi, the functional movements associated with respiration, and so forth. He will in this way necessarily soon learn to recognize the spectrum of normality and readily identify any deviation from normal, such as an immobile carina or other dysfunctional change, which signifies pathology.

No bronchoscopic examination can be considered complete unless all the bronchial openings have been identified or the reason for failure to do so determined. When difficulty arises in the identification of certain openings, a selective bronchogram can prove most helpful.

Ancillary investigative procedures, including the selective catheterization of specific segmental bronchi, will be described in a subsequent chapter.

# *Chapter 4* Dynamic Changes in the Bronchial Tree Under Conditions of Quiet Respiration or Coughing

In order to understand the changes observed in the airways, it is appropriate here to consider briefly the forces applied to the bronchial tree.

The trachea and the bronchi down to the level of the bronchioli (airways lacking a cartilaginous support structure) have a limiting membrane and a potential space surrounding their outer wall. The pressure in this potential space is a function of the intrapleural pressure. Thus, it can be stated that the volume of the larger air passages is a function of the intrapleural pressure.

During the respiratory cycle, the intrathoracic trachea and the bronchi are subjected to significant changes in volume. From total lung capacity to residual volume, the intrapulmonary airways undergo a volume change commensurate with the decrease in size of the lung as a whole, and in particular, there is a shortening of the longitudinal axis (Figs. VIII a and b). Failure of the airways to shorten

Figs. 29–56 see pp. 58–69

a

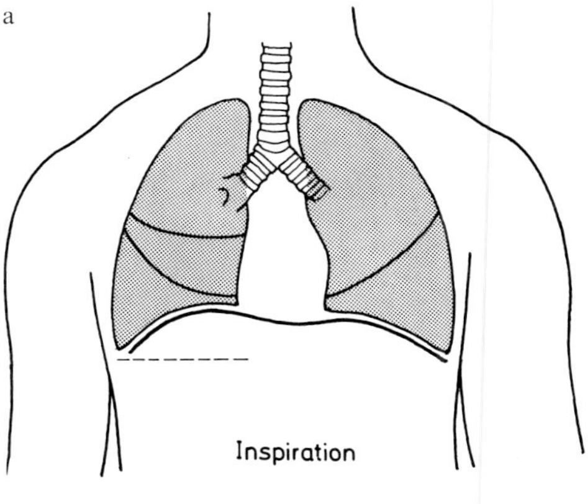


Fig. VIII. See text

b

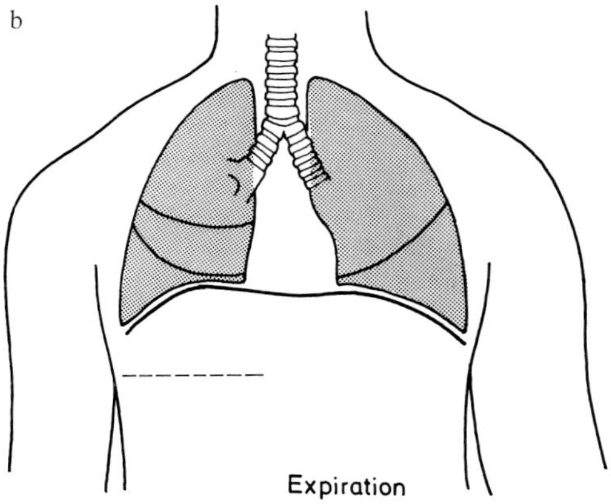


c

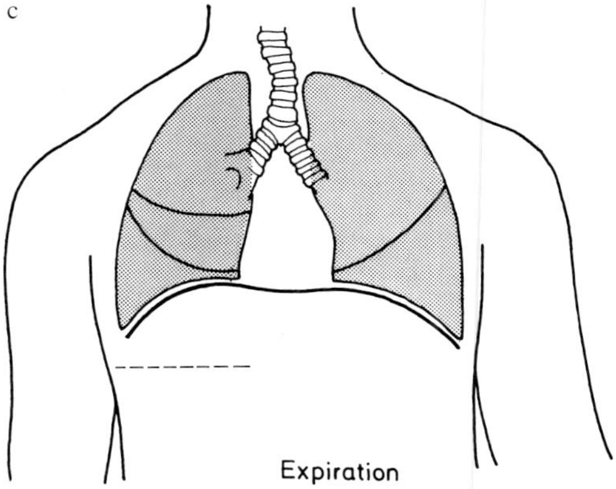

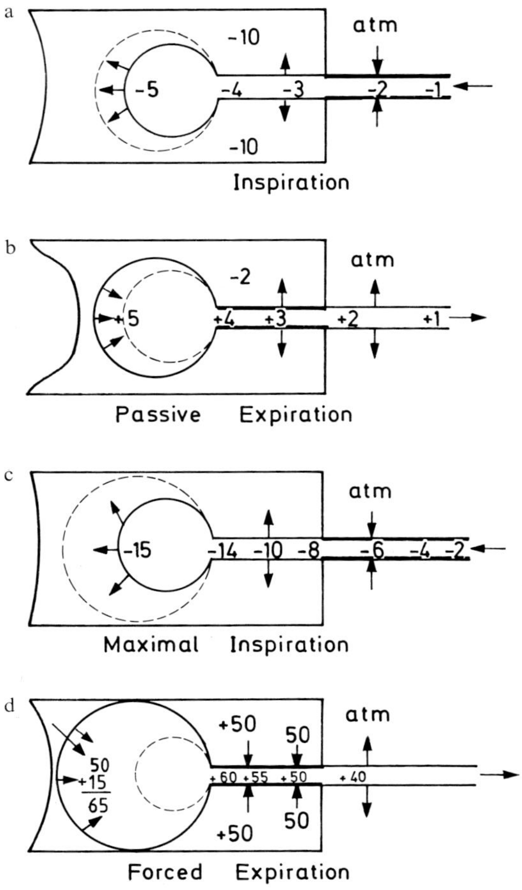


Fig. IX. See text

with diminution of lung volume produces a tendency to kinking and consequent obstruction.

During expiration, too, the carina moves at least 2 cm toward the thoracic inlet, and if the trachea does not shorten accordingly, it will fold on itself (Fig. VIIIc).

During an inspiration, the negative pressure in the thorax increases, thereby overcoming the elastic recoil of the lung and creating a negative pressure in the alveoli. Air now flows into the lungs (Fig. IXa). During this inspiratory flow, there is a subatmospheric negative pressure throughout the bronchial tree, and this becomes progressively more negative as the alveoli are approached (Fig. IXa).

This is necessarily so, since the inflow of air would otherwise be impossible. Although the pressure in the intrathoracic airways is subatmospheric, that in the pleural cavity and peribronchial spaces is even more negative. This tends to increase the internal diameter of the airways (Fig. IXa), while the increase in lung volume and the inspiratory downward movement both tend to expand the longitudinal axis of the airways.

However, while the intraluminal pressure of the extrathoracic airways also becomes negative, the surrounding pressure remains atmospheric, so that there will be forces tending to collapse the extrathoracic airways during inspiration (Fig. IXa).

Theoretically this implies that the pressure difference across the wall of the extrathoracic trachea during an inspiration will tend to narrow the lumen. In practice, however, the extrathoracic trachea is normally a relatively rigid structure resisting externally applied pressures. This is due to the cricoid, which is a complete circle of cartilage, and the supporting tracheal cartilages which have a relatively narrow posterior membrane.

During passive expiration a reversal of differential pressure relationships takes place. When the inspiratory muscles relax, the elastic recoil of the lungs favors a return to FRC (Fig. IXb). While air flow persists, the intraluminal airways pressure must of necessity exceed atmospheric pressure. A degree of negative pressure is normally maintained in the pleural cavity throughout passive expiration (Fig. IXb).

During a forced expiration, e.g., a cough, the expiratory muscles contract, and a positive pressure is created in the pleural cavity (Fig. IXd). The sum of this pressure and that exerted by the elastic recoil comprises the intra-alveolar pressure. As air is expelled from the lungs, intraluminal pressure declines progressively along the airways until a point is reached within the thorax where this pressure equals the surrounding pressure, the so-called equal pressure point. From this point towards the thoracic outlet, the intrathoracic pressure will exceed the intraluminal pressure and therefore tend to collapse the airways. This compression effect is never exerted on the extrathoracic trachea since the pressure within this structure always exceeds atmospheric pressure during expiration.

In summary then, the pressure difference across the walls of the intrathoracic airway will, during inspiration, tend to enlarge the lumen of the air passages. The reverse relationship obtains in expiration. The observed changes are accentuated during forced inspiratory and expiratory movements. Narrowing of the extrathoracic airway associated with an obstruction of the larynx or the extrathoracic trachea will be exaggerated by the increased negative pressure created within the airway during inspiration. This explains why stridor due to upper respiratory obstruction is heard mainly during inspiration. Rhonchi and wheezing related to narrowing of the intrathoracic airways are, in contrast, accentuated by expiration. Intrathoracic airway narrowing may be minimized by a shift in the equal pressure point to the exterior of the thorax.

When these mechanical changes are considered, the dynamics of the airways during respiration and coughing are readily understood, and the functional consequences of pathology can be recognized bronchoscopically.

The above effects on the large airways can be observed through the bronchoscope in a spontaneously breathing patient. During inspiration, the vocal chords open away from each other (Fig. 29), thereby reducing air flow resistance and minimizing the pressure differential between the lumen of the intrathoracic trachea and the atmosphere. During expiration, the vocal chords approach each other (Fig. 30), with a corresponding increase in airways resistance. This increase in resistance to extrathoracic air flow shifts the equal pressure point toward the thoracic outlet and thus reduces the compression effect exerted on the intrathoracic airways. Supplementation of the extrathoracic airways resistance effected by expiration through pursed lips alleviates the excessive collapse seen in pathological airways.

The cricoid cartilage, as already stated, describes a complete circle (Fig. 7c) which, together with the relatively narrow posterior openings of the cartilages comprising the extrathoracic airway, lends rigidity to the total structure (Fig. 8). The position of the cricoid cartilage relative to the thoracic inlet is not constant and depends on the degree of flexion or extension of the head and neck. The range of movement from full extension to full flexion is approximately 3 cm. Normally, the extrathoracic trachea below the cricoid is relatively short.

With the head in extension during bronchoscopy, the distance from the cricoid to the thoracic inlet extends over three vertebrae (Fig. 7a).

Volume changes in the extrathoracic airways during bronchoscopy in which a rigid instrument is employed are usually minimal and not easily demonstrated. This may be explained by the relatively low resistance to air flow through the bronchoscope in comparison with that normally encountered across the vocal chords. As the bronchoscope enters the intrathoracic portion of the trachea, however, the changes during respiration become much more obvious.

There is a wide normal variation in the space between the posterior attachments of the C-shaped cartilages, this space being spanned by the posterior membrane of the trachea (Figs. 31, 32 and 33). The width of the posterior membrane in-

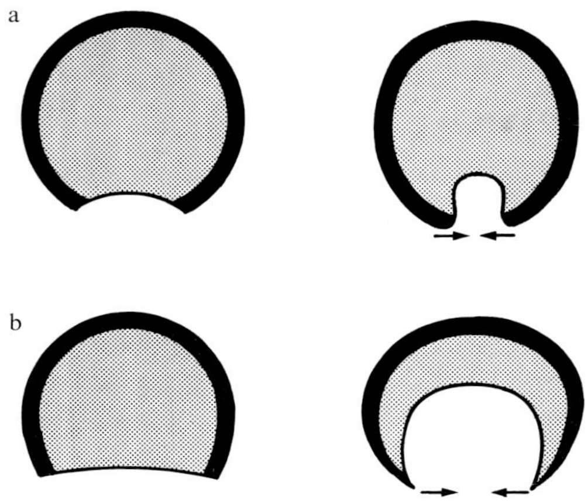


Fig. X. See text

creases towards the carina, the tracheal cartilages approaching a semicircular shape at this juncture (Fig. 34) in most individuals, although considerable variation is again observed. The same holds true for the right and left main bronchi where a semicircular cartilage structure is the rule (Fig. 35).

Normal respiration is associated with a to-and-fro movement of the posterior membrane, the latter completing a full circle with the cartilage segments during inspiration (Fig. 36) and encroaching on the lumen in expiration. A forced expiration greatly accentuates this movement. Once again, a wide normal variation dependent on many factors is observed. If bronchiolar constriction is present and the equal pressure point far to the periphery, greater prolapse of the membrane occurs than is normally seen (Fig. 37), but this can be reduced by the administration of a bronchodilator (Fig. 38).

Where the tracheal cartilages are segments of circles, the bulging of the membrane aided perhaps by smooth-muscle contraction will tend to approximate the open ends, thereby completing the circle (Figs. Xa and 37). The resultant stabilizing effect on the trachea is likely to be greater in cartilages with near complete ring structure than in tracheal segments with a wide posterior membrane (Fig. Xb and Figs. 33 and 34). The wider the posterior membrane, the greater the tendency to prolapse with increased pressure in the thoracic cavity (Fig. 39).

Posterior membrane prolapse is more pronounced at the level of the carina and in the main bronchi (Figs. 40 and 41). It is responsible for a measure of anteroposterior compression of the carina.

Anatomical structure usually has functional significance. The mobile posterior membrane is probably of functional importance during a cough. The decrease in anteroposterior diameter of the trachea and major bronchi occasioned by the inward bulge of the posterior membrane, a feature shared by subjects with normal lung mechanics as measured by existing methods, probably increases the velocity of air flow and consequently enhances the efficacy of a cough in the removal of mucus and foreign material. It may further be significant that the longitudinal mucosal corrugations, where present, are found mainly in the trachea from a level a few centimeters above the carina, in the main bronchi, and around the lobar and segmental bronchial openings. In these situations, they may serve to promote laminar flow during intraluminal prolapse of the posterior membrane.

The two main bronchi can accommodate a far greater volume than the undivided airway of the trachea, and this holds true at each stage of bronchial division. A logical assumption would be that the inspiratory air flow velocity in the major bronchi is below that in the trachea. During expiration, however, the measure of posterior membrane prolapse is relatively greater in the bronchi than in the trachea. This implies that the difference in expiratory velocity of air flow in these structures may well be minimized by the proportionately larger reduction of the lumen of the bronchi. While it is difficult to record these events by photographic means, and even more difficult to explain the mechanisms involved, one does on occasion gain the impression that membrane prolapse is propagated in wave form from beyond the carina toward the thoracic outlet, an effect calculated to facilitate the propulsion of foreign material and sputum.

The excursions of the posterior membrane and the associated shortening of the bronchial tree increase the effectiveness of the cough maneuver in the removal of secretions and foreign material from the airway. When the reduction in lumen size accounted for by posterior membrane prolapse exceeds certain limits, however, the available driving pressure becomes inadequate in the face of the consequent resistance increase, and velocity declines. Under abnormal conditions, a total collapse of the lumen beyond the equal pressure point will obstruct air flow during a forced expiratory maneuver.

## Abnormal Dynamics of the Airways

As already outlined there is considerable variation in the width of the posterior tracheobronchial membrane. The C-shaped cartilages describing relatively smaller segments of large circles are more vulnerable to any increase in extramural pressure than those cartilages forming large segments of smaller circles.

During coughing, the bronchial wall is exposed to recurrent variations in pressure. A chronic cough subjects the bronchial cartilages to a fair degree of stress over a lengthy period. This may eventually lead to sagging of the anterior tracheal wall: The author observed this at close hand in a 40-year-old woman with clinically normal lungs, who had suffered from a persistent irritant cough for two years following esophagectomy (Fig. 42).

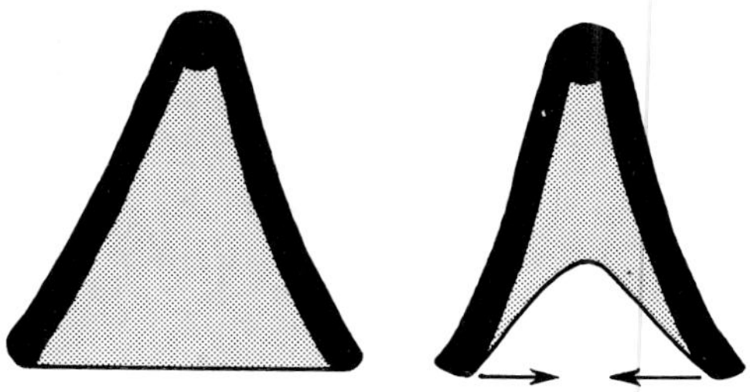

Fig. XI. See text

In chronic bronchitis a sagging and flattening of one lateral bronchial wall may be seen, or both sides may be involved (Figs. 43 and 44). When both lateral walls are affected, the tracheal cartilages assume a triangular shape (Fig. 45). These triangular cartilages are intrinsically less stable and incapable of resisting increases in intrathoracic pressure effectively. Triangular change is most liable to occur in tracheae with wide posterior membranes. The increased pressure associated with a forced expiratory maneuver results in marked bulging of the posterior membrane, and it also approximates the lateral sides of the triangle (Fig. XI). The cartilage at the apex of the triangle often displays thickening, and this probably results from the hinge effect in the modified structure. In such cases, a forced expiration may produce total occlusion of the lumen (Fig. 46).

There is a second mechanism by which the trachea or bronchi can be occluded. As has been described, the carina moves towards the thoracic outlet during expiration, necessitating longitudinal shortening of the trachea and bronchi in proportion to the reduction of lung volume in order to obviate kinking of the tubular structure (Figs. XIIa and b). The inability of the airways to shorten during expiration implies that the airways are, in practical terms, functionally too long, and they consequently tend to obstruct laterally during expiration (Fig. XIIc). Under

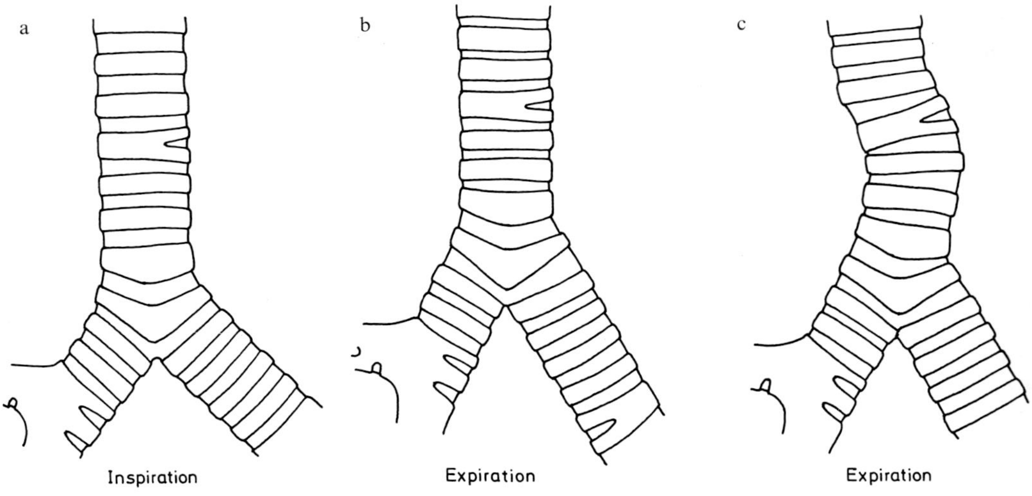


Fig. XII. See text

these circumstances, the tracheal cartilages are U-shaped and may even be obliquely orientated (Fig. 47). The posterior membrane is also relatively narrower. These appearances are often misconstrued as the consequence of extratracheal pressure exerted by tumors.

Forced expiration aggravates this deformity, and a side-to-side narrowing of the trachea occurs which may result in total occlusion (Fig. 48). This side-to-side distortion may also be seen at the level of the carina or more distally and may be accompanied by marked posterior membrane prolapse (Fig. 49).

Abnormal narrowing of the trachea and the larger airways interferes with the cough mechanism and renders it totally ineffective. This means that the drainage of secretions is impaired, thereby greatly increasing the risk of infection. This sequence of events provides an explanation of recurrent bronchial infection in patients with normal immune mechanisms and would also account for the refractory nature of respiratory infections in such patients.

The tendency to occlusion may show a predilection for one main bronchus or may afflict a number of lobar or segmental bronchi more selectively (Figs. 50, 51 or 52, 53), affording an explanation for recurrent infection of a particular lobe or bronchopulmonary segment.

## Further Use of the Bronchoscope as a Research Tool in Obstructive Airways Disease

Apart from its uses in the study and visualization of mechanical and structural change in the larger airways, the bronchoscope also permits observation of bronchospasm and associated functional change. Figures illustrate the bronchoscopic findings in a patient who underwent bronchoscopy for hemoptysis, and whose airways were known to be sensitive. With the bronchoscope in the right intermediate bronchus (Fig. 54) the bronchus just distal to the tip of the bronchoscope was stimulated mechanically. Bronchoconstriction promptly ensued and was associated with narrowing of the middle lobe bronchus and the exudation of droplets of clear fluid from the mucous membrane (Fig. 55). Following withdrawal of the bronchoscope by a few centimeters, observation over a 5–10 min period revealed the development of a secondary hyperemia and the secretion of thick, viscid mucus (Fig. 56). When reflex reactions are to be studied in this way, care must be taken to avoid the use of atropine and other anticholinergic drugs in the premedication. Minimal local anesthesia should be employed and special precautions taken to prevent spraying of the distal airways.

# *Chapter 5* Tumors

The thorax and its contents are prone to a variety of tumors, most of them malignant. These can be metastatic from areas outside the thorax, part of a general malignant condition involving several glands and the lungs, e.g., Hodgkin's disease, or arise primarily from intrathoracic organs. The most important of these malignant tumors is certainly primary cancer of the bronchus. The incidence of lung cancer is increasing at an alarming rate, and the prognosis is on the whole extremely poor. Early diagnosis and surgical removal offer the only prospect of prolonged survival.

Bronchoscopy remains the single most important investigation in establishing the diagnosis of bronchial cancer. The development of the fiberoptic bronchoscope has extended visibility to the smaller subsegmental bronchi, and has made possible the viewing of many more tumors than was previously the case.

The most important indication for bronchoscopy in the diagnosis of malignancy of the airways is the suspicion of cancer on the part of the clinician. When dealing with patients over the age of 40 years with chest symptoms, a high index of suspicion is fully justified. It may be stated that the frequency of performance of any special investigation relates directly to its availability, reliability, and ease in execution. Where clinics are endowed with good facilities, it is customary for chest physicians to conduct their own bronchoscopic examinations, and as a consequence, more such procedures are carried out here than in less well-equipped institutions. When the patient has to be referred to an endoscopy clinic for the purpose, bronchoscopy is frequently postponed and the patient followed up instead by chest radiography after two to three months. Where sufficient suspicion of malignancy is nurtured to warrant follow-up by radiographic means, there would certainly seem in most cases to be an indication for bronchoscopic investigation. An analogous situation exists where a gastroenterologist, suspecting a rectal or sigmoid cancer on digital examination of the rectum, proceeds without delay to sigmoidoscopy during this initial consultation. While the poor prognosis of bronchial cancer engenders understandable pessimism, the clinician should guard against an attitude of fatalistic inactivity. Even though the overall prognostic outlook is bleak and few patients survive longer than five years, the physician still has a duty to attempt to improve the individual patient's prognosis by whatever means at his disposal.

Bronchoscopy is indicated in all patients with suspected pulmonary tumor, even in cases of peripherally sited coin lesions where visualization of the tumor itself is improbable, even with the aid of a fiberoptic bronchoscope. Bronchial washings sampled for cytological and biochemical studies frequently yield positive results. The lesion can also be reached with a catheter, allowing a brush biopsy to be taken of the area. It is also important to perform bronchoscopy in the preoperative context to exclude any factors which might contraindicate thoracotomy, e.g., thickening and fixation of the carina

Figs. 57–99 see pp. 68–83

related to malignant infiltration of adjacent lymph nodes.

Thorough clinical and radiological assessment of the patient prior to bronchoscopy is essential. Tomography should be employed to facilitate radiological localization of the lesion where indicated. Even if a central situation of the tumor is suspected, a full range of telescopes, an angled biopsy forceps, the requisite catheters and brushes, and a 4.5-mm fiberoptic flexible bronchoscope should be on hand for the eventuality of a tumor sited beyond vision in the larger bronchi.

In the presence of acute or subacute infection of the airways associated with large quantities of mucopurulent sputum, it is advantageous first to treat the infection with an appropriate antibiotic and inhalation- and physiotherapy. A few days' delay should not significantly affect the ultimate prognosis, and the bronchoscopic examination of relatively clear airways, free from mucosal inflammation and a tendency to bleed, is of far greater diagnostic value.

When the tumor is situated in one of the main bronchi or one of their main lobar branches, the diagnosis is comparatively easy and biopsy-taking presents no problems. Moreover, even if direct visualization of the tumor is impossible, indirect evidence of malignancy, such as a thickened, immobile carina, may be present, often permitting a confident diagnosis of neoplasia. In cases where the suspected tumor is visualized, a complete bronchoscopic assessment still demands inspection of all the bronchial openings on the affected and the contralateral sides of the chest, as multicentric malignant lesions do occur. The siting of the tumor should be pinpointed and the condition and mobility of the overlying and surrounding mucous membrane, the carina, and other structures assessed with accuracy.

Where bronchoscopy is performed to investigate a pulmonary or hilar mass, careful attention should be paid to all the structures from the epiglottis downward. Unrelated benign lesions are sometimes found on the epiglottis (Fig. 57 – benign cyst) and on the vocal chords (Fig. 58 – Singers' nodes; Fig. 59a – benign papilloma between the vocal chords) which may cause changes in the timber of the voice or hoarseness and which may be confused with paralysis of the left vocal chord (Fig. 60), suggesting infiltration of the recurrent laryngeal nerve.

Hoarseness associated with intrathoracic tumors is almost always related to involvement of the left recurrent laryngeal nerve in its intrathoracic course, an anatomic feature not shared by the recurrent nerve on the right. Involvement of the latter is seen only in cases of malignant infiltration of lymph nodes at the base of the neck on the right side. Vocal chord paralyses are more readily recognized during spontaneous respiration, when immobility of the affected chord can be detected. In the course of general anesthesia where relaxants are employed, this feature can easily escape notice.

Associated chest symptoms occasionally mark the presentation of a patient with a malignant growth on the vocal chords, but the bronchoscopic diagnosis usually presents no problems (Fig. 61).

Cancer of the thyroid may infiltrate the cervical trachea. Histologically, the primary tumor can be identified in a biopsy specimen taken from the site (Fig. 62). A malignant tumor of the thyroid may also compress the trachea from side-to-side without infiltrating the wall (Fig. 63). Both infiltrating and compressing tumors of primary thyroid origin give rise to a rigid immobile trachea.

Primary cancer of the trachea is extremely rare, and primary cancer of the cervical trachea is almost unknown. Localization of the level of the tumor in the trachea is of considerable importance if tracheostomy is contemplated to relieve severe distress. The practical significance of such localization is the avoidance of an incision made in the tumor tissue or the foreknowledge that the tube will have to be advanced through the substance of the tumor. In some instances, the tumor can be localized at bronchoscopy through the recognition of an associated triangulation deformity of the cartilaginous ring structure, a feature confined to the intrathoracic trachea (Fig. 64). The light of the bronchoscope in the cervical trachea is frequently visible from the exterior in a darkened room. Where transillumination is not obvious, the level of the tumor may be determined from the outside by the passage of a needle through the suprasternal notch into the trachea, providing a useful reference marker (Fig. 65).

Occlusion of the distal end of the trachea immediately above the carina can usually be ascribed to pressure exerted by surrounding lymph nodes which have undergone malignant infiltration commonly derived from a primary tumor of the right upper lobe.

Tumors occurring in the main bronchi present no diagnostic problems (Figs. 66–69). The malignant process may totally occlude a major bronchus (Fig. 70), and the surrounding mucous membrane may be very congested and hemorrhage readily. The tumor itself may also bleed on the slightest trauma. The observer is therefore well advised to advance the bronchoscope with great care and to apply the suction nozzle gently under direct vision. While this type of bleeding never assumes dangerous proportions, it may hinder assessment of the adjoining mucous membrane and other related structures and render adequate biopsy sampling difficult.

Tumors in the openings of lobar bronchi may be easy to demonstrate (Figs. 71–73). They are, however, not infrequently less obvious (Fig. 74) and could escape notice in the presence of inflammatory changes, secretions, and bleeding. The bronchoscopist should, therefore, not be satisfied before every opening has been identified and explored with an angled bronchoscope. Inflammatory change sometimes makes this impossible, and the investigation should then be repeated after the underlying infection has been treated. Infection may also blunt the edge of the spur of an opening, but cases of malignant thickening are distinguished by the firmer consistency of the spur and its relative immobility.

Often the tumor itself cannot be visualized, but the opening to the lobe is narrowed by compression and the spur is thick and immobile (Fig. 75). A deep biopsy from this thickened spur often reveals malignancy.

Adenomata of the bronchi are relatively rare and usually present with hemoptysis or radiological evidence of lobar or segmental collapse, or both (Figs. 76–79). Biopsies taken from these tumors may occasion profuse bleeding.

## Bronchoscopic Evidence of Inoperability

A part of the purpose of bronchoscopy in malignancy of the lungs is an attempt to assess the operability of the tumor. It should immediately be stated that a large number of tumors considered operable on their bronchoscopic appearances will, in fact, prove inoperable when assessed by other criteria, such as radiological evidence of paratracheal lymph node enlargement, the involvement of the ribs in apical tumors, the presence of pleural involvement, evidence of malignant infiltration in lymph nodes removed at mediastinoscopy, the finding of distant metastasis, etc. However, in very many patients unnecessary procedures and/or surgery can be avoided if a thorough bronchoscopic assessment is made.

Bronchoscopic signs of inoperability include:

1. A vocal chord paralysis, indicative of infiltrating disease involving the recurrent laryngeal nerve (Fig. 60).

2. Evidence that enlarged paratracheal lymph nodes are exerting pressure on the trachea and impairing its mobility.

3. The presence of tumors which primarily involve the trachea (Fig. 64) or have spread up its lateral wall from beyond the carina (Fig. 67).

4. Demonstrable involvement of nodes around the carina. The normal carina is sharp and has a narrow base both anteriorly and posteriorly. It is normally mobile, and transmitted pulsations of the heart are easily discerned. The carina also moves during respiration and is readily displaced laterally by the tip of the rigid bronchoscope. Infection may blunt the edge of the carina, but it remains mobile. Malignant infiltration from adjacent lymph nodes causes a thickening of the carina with a propensity to involve the anterior margin (Figs. 80 and 81). The carina also becomes relatively fixed and immobile, and a needle biopsy taken here often yields positive results. The posterior membrane may be forced into the tracheal

a

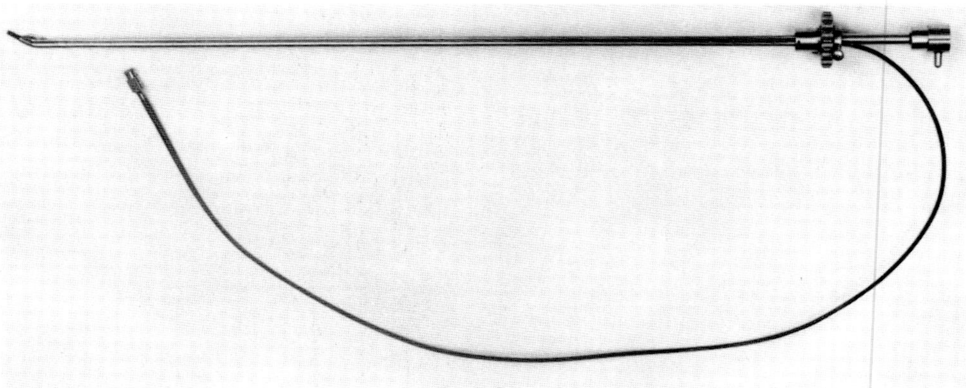

b

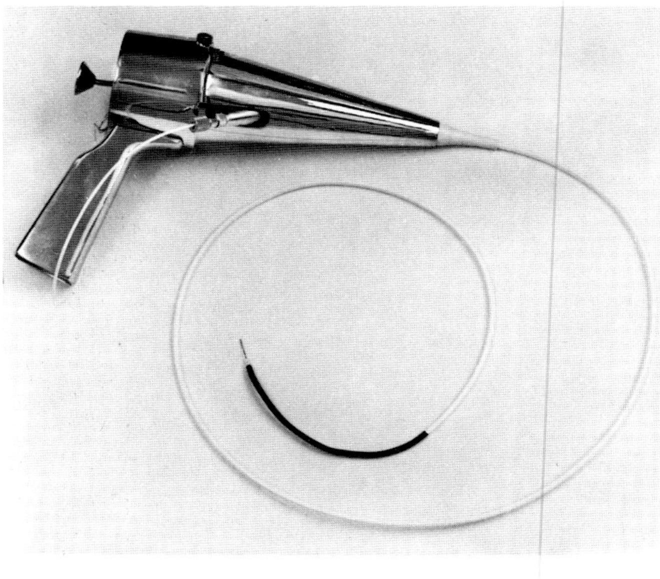

Fig. XIII. (a) Storz catheter introducer and telescopic guide for the manipulation of a catheter into lobar or segmental bronchi under vision. (b) Medi-Tech Selector Catheter for selective segmental bronchial catheterization

lumen at the level of the carina by lymph node infiltration involving the latter (Fig. 82). A relatively small tumor sited more distally is sometimes found in association with the malignant involvement of the carina (Fig. 83).

5. Extensive lymphangitic and nodal infiltration as inferred from the finding of a thickened spur of the upper lobe bronchus in association with tumors of the lower lobe (Figs. 84 and 85).

6. Thickened, edematous mucous membrane assuming longitudinal mucosal folds which simulate the normal mucosal corrugations and which extend upwards in the bronchus, being associated with peribronchial lymphatic involvement. A biopsy of these folds is often positive (Fig. 86).

When an alveolar-cell carcinoma is suspected from the radiological appearances, bronchial washings may yield positive cytological results. A histological diagnosis may be reached through direct lung biopsy sampling via the bronchoscope. The biopsy scissors are wedged in a segmental bronchus, usually one of the basal or middle lobe segmental bronchi. Biopsies sampled in this manner are frequently diagnostic (Figs. 87 and 88), and the amount of hemorrhage is usually negligible. This method of transbronchial lung biopsy may also be used in the investigation of other forms of diffuse lung disease. In cases of peripherally sited tumor, the fiberoptic bronchoscope, particularly the 4.5-mm gauge instrument, holds definite advantages in terms of biopsy technique. Under direct vision and with the aid of fluoroscopic screening, a peripherally sited lesion may be sampled by means of the brush biopsy technique. Cournand cardiac catheters may be guided under direct vision into almost any segmental bronchus (Figs. 89 and 90a) making use of a special attachment mounted on the Storz bronchoscope (Fig. XIII a). The catheter tip can also be manipulated under fluoroscopic control into the tumor area, where a brush biopsy sample may be obtained. A special catheter which facilitates manipulation is also available (Fig. XIII b). This catheter can also be introduced into any segment as required (Figs. 90b and c), and it has matching brushes. Biochemical analysis of the lysosomal enzyme activity of bronchial washings provides the basis of yet another significant diagnostic test. This technique may serve to indicate malignant disease in certain instances where cytological scrutiny has yielded negative results [5].

# *Chapter 6* Trauma of the Airways

The bronchoscope is an essential piece of equipment in the respiratory intensive care ward, and bronchoscopic evaluation is often indicated in the management of the severely injured patient.

It is sound policy to perform bronchoscopy in all patients with chest injuries for the treatment of which intermittent positive pressure respiration is indicated. The purpose of such examination is not only to exclude rupture of a bronchus but also to remove secretions and blood clot from the airways. Late complications, such as infection and lobar or segmental collapse, are kept to a minimum by this procedure. Severe or persistent hemoptysis, pneumothorax, or bronchopleural fistulae in the injured patient are absolute indications for bronchoscopy, in order to exclude the possibility of bronchial laceration.

It may at times prove extremely difficult or impossible to pass an endotracheal tube in a patient with severe injuries to the face and upper airways. Under these circumstances, it is easier and safer to pass a bronchoscope under direct vision, followed by tracheostomy while the patient is being ventilated through the bronchoscope.

Attempts by an inexperienced operator to pass an endotracheal tube under difficult circumstances may result in severe injuries to the larynx. It is possible, for instance, to avulse the anterior wall of the larynx immediately in front of the vocal chords, and the resultant collapse may occlude the opening between the chords (Fig. 91). In such cases, the tip of the bronchoscope may be employed to elevate the collapsed wall, displacing it anteriorly and permitting further passage of the instrument between the vocal chords. On occasion, a disorientated patient may pull out an endotracheal tube with the cuff still inflated, and the resultant hematoma and edema of the vocal chords may give rise to severe airways obstruction (Fig. 92). Here again a bronchoscope can be passed between the vocal chords under direct vision and without causing further trauma. An intralaryngeal tube left in position for too long is liable to cause necrosis of the vocal chords (Fig. 93), and the healing process leads to scar formation.

Lacerations of the bronchi are relatively uncommon and are usually found in the main bronchi near the carina. The carina itself may also be involved in the tear. In Fig. 94 a tear just above the opening of the right upper lobe bronchus is shown. Suturing of these lacerations may be complicated by infection, with breakdown of the suture-line resulting in a bronchopleural fistula (Fig. 95). The removal of sutures through the bronchoscope sometimes promotes healing. Granulomatous tissue forming on suture lines may also be removed via the bronchoscope, and the area may be cauterized with silver nitrate (a 25% solution applied on a pledget of cotton wool) with excellent results.

Tracheostomy is a minor surgical procedure, but it involves a major responsibility on the part of the physician and the nursing staff involved. Not infre-

Figs. 91–108 see pp. 82–89

quently, the patient, having been treated successfully by tracheostomy for an acute condition, is left with a relatively severe complication, namely tracheal stenosis or more rarely a tracheoesophageal fistula. The author believes that judicious and timely inspection of the upper airways can contribute to the prevention of these complications. When blood-tinged mucus is aspirated from the tracheostomy tube, bronchoscopic examination may reveal an ulcer at the base of the carina caused by a tracheostomy tube which is too long, or an area of sloughing and surrounding inflammation provoked by excessive or too lengthy inflation of the cuff (Fig. 96). It is this sloughing of the posterior membrane which may lead to a tracheoesophageal fistula (Fig. 97). In the author's experience of more than 1500 tracheostomies for intermittent positive pressure respiration observed over a period of 12 years, this complication was encountered only in the presence of severe secondary infection and is fortunately rare.

Stenosis of the trachea is probably the commonest complication of tracheostomy. Injury to the cricoid cartilage in particular almost invariably results in stenosis and should therefore be avoided.

Two types of stenosis of the trachea can be distinguished:

1. Injury of the tracheal rings themselves, resulting in a thickening and constriction of the tracheal wall. This stenosis may involve a segment of more than 1 cm in width and is usually located at the site of the original incision, this being demonstrated by the insertion of a needle through the tracheostomy scar (Fig. 98).

2. A membranous narrowing of the trachea is frequently seen in association with normal tracheal rings up to the margins of the stenotic area. Closer inspection reveals that the trachea immediately distal to the stenosis is again relatively normal (Fig. 99). This membranous stenosis is in fact not at the site of the tracheostomy but is located lower down towards the carina. Once again the level can be pinpointed by the insertion of a needle through the tracheostomy scar (Fig. 100). The site of this stenosis corresponds to the area occupied by the inflated cuff of the tracheostomy tube. The membrane probably forms through the organization of papillomatous outgrowths arising in the affected area, most likely in response to irritation by the cuff or associated infection. Numerous papillomas may form (Fig. 101) which later coalesce to constitute a membrane. Larger papillomatous outgrowths may similarly arise circumferentially in the trachea (Fig. 102) and eventually organize into a fibrous membrane which narrows the lumen.

Distortion of the cartilaginous contour at the site of the tracheostomy with membranous narrowing lower down is sometimes observed. In such cases a combination of mechanisms is probably involved (Fig. 103).

The only effective treatment for the first type of stenosis is excision of the stenotic segment, since dilatation is not possible. The membranous type of stenosis may, on the other hand, be treated effectively by dilatation through the bronchoscope. This is of practical significance, since the frequent intrathoracic location of this variety of tracheal stenosis renders excision far more difficult from the technical aspect.

A specially designed tracheoscope (Storz) with smooth walls and prismatic illumination from the rear as employed in the bronchoscopy of infants, also incorporating transilluminable hollow dilators, is available (Fig. XIVa). The use of this instrument permits dilatation of the stenotic area under direct vision without respiratory embarrassment. When the membrane is relatively thick and the central opening very small, lateral incision from the lumen can be effected by a ring electric-wire cautery prior to the insertion of

Fig. XIV. (a) The smooth-walled Storz tracheoscope, incorporating transilluminable hollow dilators in graded sizes, for use in the dilatation of membranous tracheal stenoses. (b) The Storz cotton carrier with spiral tip employed in the chemical cauterization of tracheal granuloma

a

b

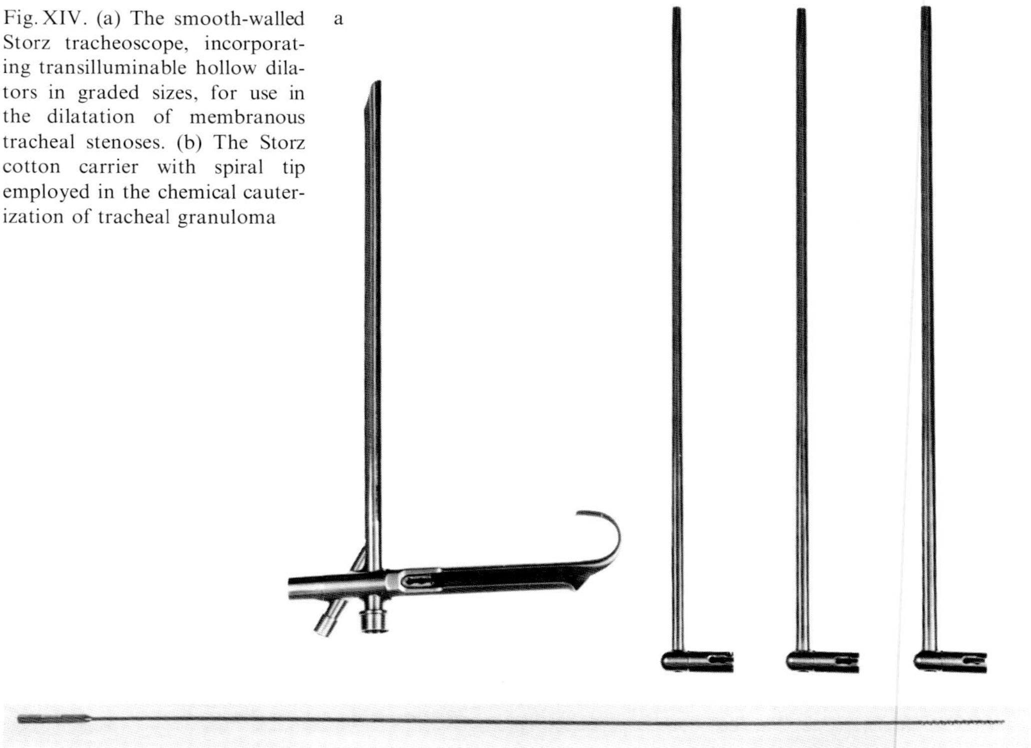

the dilator (Figs. 104 and 105). Dissected portions of the membrane may be extracted with a biopsy forceps. The results of this procedure are gratifying (Fig. 106). Where intratracheal granulomas re-form (Figs. 107 and 108), they are readily removed through the bronchoscope, and the affected area may be cauterized with 25% silver nitrate solution on a cotton pledget attached to a special cotton carrier (Fig. XIV b) (STORZ). When foreign bodies remain in the airways for some time, chronic irritation may give rise to granulation tissue which can be dealt with as described above.

# *Chapter 7* Bronchial Lavage and Postoperative Lobar and Segmental Collapse of the Lungs

Where significant quantities of secretions are produced in the airways, their efficient removal is essential if the formation of thick mucous plugs leading to segmental or lobar obstruction and collapse (Fig. 109) is to be prevented. These secretions may also become infected and, in the process of transition to mucopurulent or frankly purulent sputum sometimes lead on to acute infective tracheobronchitis, bronchopneumonia, or both. These complications are far more likely to arise where the cough mechanism is impaired in association with obstructive airways disease and especially with collapsing airways. Following abdominal or thoracic surgery, suppression of the cough maneuver by pain and/or the cough reflex by morphine and related drugs may lead to respiratory complications. The author's experience in a 1600-bed teaching hospital has been that most patients who developed postoperative lung collapse had a history of preoperative sputum production. The treatment of postoperative lung complications should therefore be viewed as primarily preventive in nature, embracing inhalation and physiotherapy preoperatively and in the immediate postoperative phase.

The effective pretreatment of any patient producing a purulent sputum is mandatory where elective surgery is planned. However, when postoperative bronchopneumonia and/or lobar or segmental collapse occur despite vigorous physiotherapy, bronchoscopy with bronchial lavage can contribute greatly to a speedy recovery and a shortened hospital stay for the patient.

An immediate reexpansion of a collapsed lobe or lung seldom results from the clearance of mucous plugs and secretions from the larger airways alone. Supplementary bronchial lavage with normal saline solution at 37° C is required. It is also essential that the patient should cough during bronchoscopy, and the employment of general anesthesia with or without relaxation consequently renders the procedure ineffective and may prove hazardous. All that is required is a limited local anesthesia of the mouth and oropharynx, with intravenous diazepam (Valium) as a useful adjunct. In a severely ill or comatose patient, minimal anesthesia may be required. Lavage is effected by the injection of 20 ml of saline through the bronchoscope, which is then sucked out. A specially designed double-lumen catheter allowing saline injection and simultaneous suction (Fig. XV) can also be used. The process is repeated 5–10 times, as required. It is necessary to administer oxygen through the side arm of the bronchoscope during the procedure. In the poor-risk patient, the lungs must be lavaged one at a time.

A collapsed lobe or entire lung contributes nothing to respiration, and any discussion of the possible hazards of bronchial lavage in such an affected lung following initial removal of the occluding plug is therefore irrelevant. The reexpansion of the lung under these conditions can only serve to improve function and the blood-gas status at the time of the procedure and subsequently, as was the

Figs. 109–132 see pp. 88–97

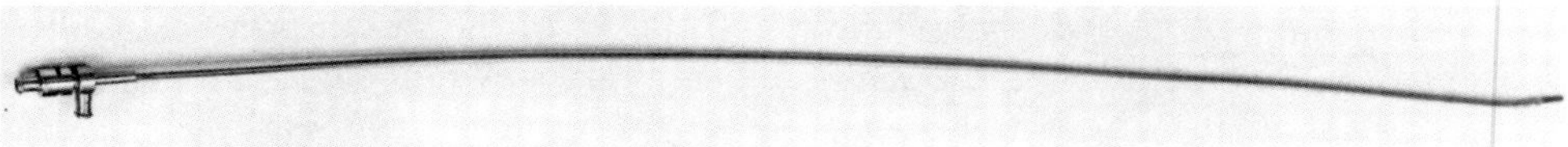

Fig. XV. Double-lumen catheter for bronchial lavage, permitting simultaneous saline injection and suction (De Kock catheter—Storz)

Table 1. $PO_2$*

| | A | B | C | D | E |
|---|---|---|---|---|---|
| 1. | 93 | 107 | 126 | 250 | 81 |
| 2. | 89 | 77 | 93 | 90 | 82 |
| 3. | 95 | 121 | 119 | 119 | 83 |
| 4. | 84 | 86 | 81 | 170 | 66 |
| 5. | 93 | 97 | 95 | 193 | 80 |
| 6. | 78 | 106 | 94 | 160 | 69 |
| 7. | | | 108 | 180 | 79 |
| 8. | 71 | | 131 | 130 | 74 |
| 9. | 97 | | 141 | 338 | 75 |
| 10. | 106 | 100 | 78 | 79 | 85 |
| Average | 89 | 99 | 104 | 170 | 77 |

* Columns B, C, and D express values recorded during oxygen administration via the side inlet port of the bronchoscope

Table 2. $PCO_2$

| | A | B | C | D | E |
|---|---|---|---|---|---|
| 1. | 43 | 59 | 48 | 45 | 36 |
| 2. | 35 | 43 | 43 | 37 | 34 |
| 3. | 24 | 30 | 28 | 28 | 20 |
| 4. | 35 | 40 | 37 | 44 | 37 |
| 5. | 32 | 37 | 37 | 41 | 38 |
| 6. | 33 | 45 | 50 | 50 | 51 |
| 7. | | | 21 | 44 | 35 |
| 8. | 44 | | 34 | 33 | 32 |
| 9. | 40 | | 46 | 41 | 39 |
| 10. | 31 | 36 | 43 | 42 | 39 |
| Average | 35 | 41 | 39 | 38 | 36 |

Table 3. pH

| | A | B | C | D | E |
|---|---|---|---|---|---|
| 1. | 7.42 | 7.31 | 7.35 | 7.35 | 7.34 |
| 2. | 7.39 | 7.30 | 7.25 | 7.25 | 7.40 |
| 3. | 7.52 | 7.36 | 7.32 | 7.32 | 7.48 |
| 4. | 7.39 | 7.26 | 7.31 | 7.25 | 7.34 |
| 5. | 7.42 | 7.36 | 7.36 | 7.32 | 7.38 |
| 6. | 7.41 | 7.36 | 7.30 | 7.28 | 7.34 |
| 7. | | | 7.39 | 7.40 | 7.40 |
| 8. | 7.12 | | 7.25 | 7.28 | 7.33 |
| 9. | 7.41 | | 7.34 | 7.33 | 7.36 |
| 10. | 7.39 | 7.41 | 7.35 | 7.32 | 7.34 |
| Average | 7.39 | 7.33 | 7.32 | 7.31 | 7.37 |

case in the patients illustrated in Figures 110–117.

Viscid secretions may similarly be removed by means of this technique. Provided that care is taken not to suppress the cough reflex and the patient does cough during the procedure, no significant respiratory embarrassment occurs, as may be inferred from the measurement of the arterial $PO_2$ (Table 1), $PCO_2$ (Table 2), and pH (Table 3) prior to bronchoscopy (A), immediately preceding bronchial lavage (B), during the procedure itself (C), and at subsequent intervals of 10 min (D) and 20 min (E). Representative values obtained in 10 patients at the stated intervals are set out in Tables 1–3. The enhanced arterial oxygen tensions recorded in columns B, C, and D of Table 1 reflect the continuous supply of free-flowing oxygen entering through the side inlet port of the bronchoscope. The values entered in column E are those recorded following the cessation of oxygen supplementation. The mean $PO_2$ level determined at this stage registers a slight but definite decrease in respect of the mean control value shown in column A, and this discrepancy can be explained in terms of a measure of alveolar collapse precipitated by the penetration of a small quantity of the lavage fluid to the level of the respiratory bronchioles, and by the temporary removal of the alveolar nitrogen "cushion" through the injection of oxygen at concentrations greatly in excess of atmospheric. The consequent near-complete absorption by diffusion of the alveolar gaseous contents results in atelectasis which persists until alveolar nitrogen tension is restored and intra-alveolar fluid absorbed or expelled, a sequence which usually occurs rapidly.

Frequently, but not invariably, a mucopurulent plug can be located in the airway corresponding to the collapsed area, and its removal by bronchial lavage may result in reexpansion of the lung, as illustrated by the following: collapse of the left lung due to occlusion of the left main bronchus (Figs. 110–112), collapse of the right lower lobe (Figs. 113 and 114), where the inflamed but still patent middle lobe opening can be seen; obstruction of the right intermediate bronchus with collapse of the right lower and middle lobes (Figs. 115–117). The thickened, inflamed spurs of nonobstructed bronchial openings can be seen in adjacent areas of the lung.

Not infrequently no definite plug can be demonstrated despite the presence of large quantities of mucopurulent secretions. In a proportion of cases of total lung collapse reexpansion immediately follows bronchial lavage (Figs. 118 and 119; 120 and 121), even though bronchoscopy had failed to reveal an occlusive plug.

Collapse of the right upper lobe is frequently seen in patients, especially children, during intermittent positive pressure respiration via a tracheostomy. More often than not this can be treated successfully with physiotherapy or bronchoscopy with lavage, or both. Where the collapse persists despite active treatment, the affected upper lobe bronchus may be catheterized and the lobe irrigated with good effect, as shown in Figures 122–124.

Bronchoscopy with selective catheterization of the bronchus draining the affected lobe may be successful in treating a lung abscess. The sequence of illustrations (Figs. 125–132) outlines the procedure in one such patient. This was a 75-year-old male, severely ill and toxemic as a result of an abscess in the right middle lobe (Figs. 125 and 126). On bronchoscopic examination, the right middle lobe bronchial opening was found to be occluded and inflamed (Fig. 127). A catheter was passed through this opening (Fig. 128) and a large quantity of pus drained. The drainage of pus from the opening continued after withdrawal of the catheter, the orifice itself remaining patent (Fig. 129). This procedure was followed by a remarkable clinical improvement which was paralleled by shrinkage of the abscess area demonstrated on chest radiography three days later (Fig. 130). A selective bronchogram at an interval of two months revealed bronchiectasis and parenchymal destruction of the afflicted middle lobe (Figs. 131 and 132).

# *Chapter 8* Tuberculosis Involving the Airways

Although bronchoscopy is seldom if ever invoked as a means of establishing the diagnosis of pulmonary tuberculosis, the extent and severity of bronchial involvement in tuberculosis can be assessed only through a bronchoscopic study of the airways.

The associated lymph node enlargement, which is a characteristic feature of primary tuberculosis, may produce distortion and narrowing of the bronchial lumen (Fig. 133). Total occlusion, particularly of the right middle lobe bronchus, is liable to occur (Figs. 134 and 135). A tuberculous lymph node may erode the bronchial mucous membrane, giving rise to a tumor-like mass protruding into the lumen (Fig. 136).

Enlarged tuberculous nodes surrounding the origin of lobar bronchi can result in a thickening and fixation of the spur of the opening, producing an effect not dissimilar to that of a malignant process (Figs. 137 and 138).

Healed intrabronchial tuberculosis may encompass fibrotic narrowing of a bronchus with resultant collapse and bronchiectasis of the lobe or segments distal to the lesion (Figs. 139 and 140). The healed tuberculous process may produce localized stenosis of a single lobar bronchus, e.g., that of the middle lobe (Fig. 141), or result in an associated distortion of the right main bronchus (Fig. 142).

Cavitating tuberculosis with heavily infected sputum may rarely be associated with caseating tuberculosis of the larynx and trachea (Figs. 143–145). The epiglottis may become swollen and edematous (Fig. 143), while the glottis and vocal chords may virtually be destroyed by the caseating process (Fig. 144). The trachea and carina may also be involved by the caseating tuberculous process (Fig. 145).

Figs. 133–147 see pp. 96–101

## Primary Amyloid Disease of the Airways

This condition is illustrated by the following case history. A 48-year-old medical practitioner presented with a history of episodic slight wheezing over some years and repeated hemoptysis of recent onset. Clinical and radiological examination of the chest revealed no abnormalities. On bronchoscopic examination the mucous membrane of the trachea appeared abnormally thick. The carina displayed an irregular, nodular surface but was quite mobile (Fig. 146). In the left main bronchus at the level of the upper lobe bronchus, a dark cherry-red mass was seen which all but occluded the lumen (Fig. 147).

Biopsy examination of the tumor and of the nodules on the carina disclosed the histological appearances of amyloid. Serum protein electrophoresis, tests of renal and liver function, the erythrocyte sedimentation rate, and a biopsy examination of rectal mucous membrane demonstrated no abnormality, and the diagnosis of primary amyloid disease was made. Resection of the tumor mass obstructing the left main bronchus was performed through the bronchoscope, and no local recurrence was observed over a six-year follow-up period. The patient remains free of symptoms.

# *Chapter 9* The Normal Mucous Membrane and Inflammatory Changes

Bronchoscopy seldom has as its main object the study of the bronchial mucous membrane. Information on the status of the mucous membrane is usually acquired coincidentally during the course of bronchoscopic examination on other grounds. This situation will, however, change considerably as physicians adopt a more functional orientation towards bronchoscopy. Whereas in the past the investigation of the mucous membrane was confined to cytological studies in pursuit of malignant change employing bronchial washings, biochemical and immunologic studies have now been superadded (KÜHN and DE KOCK, 1975).

If the mucous membrane is to be studied in its own right, special care should be exercised to avoid all forms of irritation, and to this end the use of a suction apparatus should be avoided if at all possible. An apparently normal mucous membrane may lose its delicate pink appearance following a bout of coughing in a sensitive patient and assume a reddened, indurated appearance. Suction or other forms of mechanical stimulation may similarly bring about almost instantaneous change in the mucous membrane (Figs. 54–56). By the same token, coughing immediately prior to the bronchoscopic examination is certain to affect the amount of hyperemia which is subsequently noted. It is therefore advisable to inspect the mucous membrane as an initial procedure, since any description of erythematous or edematous change based on the membrane appearance on completion of bronchoscopy will be of little diagnostic value.

The normal bronchial mucosa is usually pink (Figs. 8 and 9) and thin, and delicate superficial blood vessels are often seen. The color of the membrane is, however, subject to great variation, and this impression is accentuated by the infinite nuances imparted by varying photographic techniques, implicit in the type of film used, the nature of the light source, exposure time, and the processing method employed. The color documented in a photograph can therefore at best only represent an approximation of the true color of the mucosa.

Longitudinal mucosal corrugations caused by hypertrophied elastic connective tissue bundles are frequently observed in the posterior membranous wall of the lower trachea and the main bronchi. These corrugations may remain prominent up to the limits of bronchoscopic visibility (Fig. 148). If structural changes are assumed usually to have functional significance, it seems reasonable to postulate that these corrugations promote laminar air flow, and that this might be of special import when, during a forced expiration, the posterior membrane prolapses into the lumen of the airway (see Chapt. 4).

Present knowledge does not permit acceptable classification of bronchitis on the basis of bronchoscopically observed mucosal change. The more commonly occurring changes are demonstrated in Figures 149–159, and the author's views as to their possible significance are presented in the accompanying text.

---

Figs. 148–159 see pp. 102–105

A granulomatous appearance of the mucosa is often seen in bronchitis, and the membrane is overlain by fragmented particles of purulent mucus (Fig. 149). Bacteriological culture of these secretions usually yields negative results. This is the appearance which is frequently peculiar to heavy cigarette smokers and patients labeled with the clinical diagnosis of chronic bronchitis.

Acute bronchitis, on the other hand, is characterized by a reddened, swollen mucous membrane (Fig. 150) which occasions a blunting of the spurs of the lobar bronchial openings (Fig. 151). The swelling of the mucous membrane and the associated mucopurulent secretions may narrow the bronchial lumen to such an extent (Fig. 152) that they contribute to overall bronchial obstruction in relation to bronchospasm.

In chronic bronchitis with atrophy of the mucous membrane, superimposed acute infection may provoke acute inflammatory changes but relatively slight secretions (Fig. 153).

Alternatively, a pale yellow mucosa with membranous purulent secretions may result (Fig. 154). Where chronic bronchitis is marked by prolonged severe coughing, the characteristic findings are those of an erythematous, indurated membrane clothing the structurally distorted cartilages already described (see Chapt. 4, Figs. 45–48).]

Chronic bronchitis and emphysema may also be associated with an atrophic mucous membrane in which the dilated openings of distended submucosal glands are visible (Figs. 155–157).

Although no distinct abnormalities can usually be identified on bronchoscopic examination of patients with bronchiectasis, it may be possible to demonstrate fibrosis and distortion of the mucous membrane in the presence of severely disrupted bronchial architecture (Figs. 158 and 159).

# *Chapter 10* Bronchography via the Bronchoscope

A detailed commentary on bronchographic indications and technique is not within the scope of this book, nor does the author wish to suggest that bronchography via the bronchoscope is the method of choice. However, indications for bronchoscopy and bronchography frequently coexist in the individual patient. The need for selective bronchography may moreover arise during the conduct of a bronchoscopic examination supplemented by fiberoptic endoscopy, when negative findings dictate the use of contrast media to reach a definitive diagnosis or to guide the surgeon in his operative approach. An entirely adequate bronchogram can be obtained under these circumstances, provided that bronchial filling with contrast media is undertaken under direct fluoroscopic control (Figs. 160 and 161). Care must be taken to direct local anesthetic spray down both main bronchi, since any spillage of contrast media into the contralateral bronchus from that which is being filled selectively may otherwise provoke coughing. The selectivity of the injection is ensured through the use of a catheter guided into position via the bronchoscope.

Marked narrowing of a main bronchus may preclude distal inspection. The use of contrast media may here serve to outline the extent of the stenosis and reveal whether the distal lobes are normal or not (Fig. 162).

Filling of the bronchi may sometimes prove slow and inadequate where the patient's breathing is shallow. Here the Sanders injector may be used to propel the contrast media distally and fill the entire bronchial tree by dispersion. This technique clearly demarcates the normal and abnormal areas (Figs. 163 and 164).

On bronchoscopic inspection, the right middle lobe bronchial opening in a patient with suspected middle lobe pathology may appear normal. A bronchogram performed at the time of the study may then reveal patent but abnormal bronchi (Fig. 165).

The case of a child who accidentally inhaled sulphuric acid further illustrates the usefulness of this approach. Bronchoscopic assessment was hindered by numerous areas of stenosis in the trachea and major bronchi which had been caused by residual fibrosis, and here a simultaneous bronchogram proved essential for anatomical orientation and in the determination of the extent of distal injury (Figs. 166 and 167).

A limited selective bronchogram is frequently indicated. Localization of the contrast media is readily achieved through placement of a cardiac Swan-Ganz catheter in the relevant lobar or segmental bronchial orifice, employing the Storz catheter deflector under direct telescopic vision. The distal balloon on the catheter is inflated under vision until it occludes the bronchial opening. A 2% solution of xylocaine (lidocaine) is then injected through the main lumen of the catheter, preliminary to filling the bronchi with contrast media (Figs. 168–172).

A further application of this form of selective bronchography is illustrated by the case of a patient who underwent bron-

Figs. 160–182 see pp. 106–113

choscopic examination on account of a mass in the right hilum. Inspection showed the right upper lobar opening to be compressed and its spur thickened. The fiberoptic bronchoscope could not be passed into the upper lobe bronchus, whereas a Swan-Ganz catheter was easily positioned for selective bronchography which failed to demonstrate filling of the anterior segment of the upper lobe (Fig. 173). Following deflation of the balloon, contrast media was injected intermittently while the catheter was cautiously withdrawn.

The main right upper lobe bronchus was filled segmentally, and the site of the obstruction could therefore be pinpointed (Fig. 174). An angled biopsy scissors was passed to the pathologic area and a biopsy sample taken. Histological examination showed a well-differentiated squamous-cell carcinoma. Subsequent filling of the right main bronchus with contrast media revealed an indentation ascribed to protrusion of an infiltrated lymph node (Fig. 174). It was also noted that the apical segment of the lower lobe and the entire middle lobe failed to fill with contrast media. When the bronchoscope was advanced into the intermediate bronchus, satisfactory filling of the apical segment of the lower lobe was accomplished (Fig. 175), but middle lobe filling remained inadequate. Once again the Swan-Ganz catheter was utilized for selective catheterization with localized bronchography, and this maneuver resulted in a normal selective bronchogram of the middle lobe (Fig. 176).

When a peripheral pulmonary lesion has been visualized with the fiberoptic bronchoscope, its exact location can be determined by means of selective bronchography (Figs. 177 and 178).

Conventional methods frequently fail to outline an abscess cavity with contrast media, but selective catheterization of the affected segment may achieve this and prove useful in demonstrating the size of the cavity (Figs. 179 and 180).

Not infrequently, an adult patient may present the radiologic features of a completely destroyed lung in the absence of any appreciable pulmonary complaints or history of chronic disease. In such cases, bronchoscopic examination may reveal an apparently normal mucous membrane with little or no evidence of chronic inflammation. During forced expiration or coughing, the major bronchi remain patent, although a normal degree of luminal narrowing may be present. Bronchography, on the other hand, may show extensive bronchiectasis during inspiration (Fig. 181), while an overall narrowing down and associated emptying of the dilated airways takes place in the course of a forced expiration or cough (Fig. 182). This means that the patient can, with relative ease, clear the affected lung of contrast media. Effective drainage of this nature probably explains the fact that remarkably few symptoms and little evidence of infection are observed in respect of what is certainly a grossly abnormal lung. (See also Abnormal Dynamics of the Airways, Chapt. 4.)

# *References*


1. Stradling, P.: Diagnostic bronchoscopy: An introduction, 2nd ed. Edinburgh and London: Churchill Livingstone, 1973.
2. Ikeda, S.: Atlas of flexible bronchofiberscopy. Tokyo: Igaku Shoin, Ltd., 1974.
3. Sanders, R.D.: Two ventilating attachments for bronchoscopes. Delaware Med. J. **39**, 170 (1967)
4. Keller, R., Waldvogel, H., and Herzog, H.: Neurolept analgesia for bronchoscopic examinations. Chest **67**, 315 (1975).
5. Kühn, S.H. and De Kock, M.A.: A preliminary study of elevated alkaline phosphatase and cathepsin in bronchial aspirates of patients with lung cancer and bronchitis. Chest **68**, 326 (1975).
6. Albertini, R.E., Harrell, J.H., and Moser, K.M.: Management of arterial hypoxemia induced by fiberoptic bronchoscopy. Chest **67**, 134 (1975).
7. Nahas, H.C.: Bronchoscopy and its complications. Leb. Med. J. **27**, 609 (1974).
8. Lampton, L.M.: Bronchofiberscopy: Caution! J. Amer. med. Assoc. **231**, 138 (1975).
9. Lett, Z.: Anesthesia for flexible fiberoptic bronchoscopy. Anesthesia **29**, 623 (1974).
10. Scheinhorn, D.J., Joyner, L.R., and Whitcomb, M.E.: Transbronchial forceps lung biopsy through the fiberoptic bronchoscope in pneumocystis carinii pneumonia. Chest **66**, 294 (1974).
11. Laurence, B.P. and Sanderson, D.R.: Anesthesia for prolonged bronchoscopy. Ann. thorac. Surg. **19**, 248 (1975).
12. Murphy, W.M. and Komorowski, R.A.: An expanded role for bronchial brushings in respiratory disease. Amer. Rev. respir. Dis. **110**, 360 (1974).
13. Sackner, M.A.: Bronchofiberscopy. Amer. Rev. respir. Dis. **111**, 62 (1973).

*Illustrations*

1a, b Epiglottis with the base of the tongue lying anteriorly. *1* Uvula; *2* tongue

2a, b Root of the tongue with epiglottis. *1* Epiglottis; *2* base of tongue

3a–c The glottis and the entrance to the larynx. The base of the epiglottis can be seen anteriorly. The level of the bronchoscope in this position, in the extended neck and in relation to the thoracic inlet, is shown in Fig. 3a. (*Cl* Clavicle); *1* base of epiglottis; *2* left vocal chord; *3* right aryepiglottic fold; *4* right corniculate tubercle

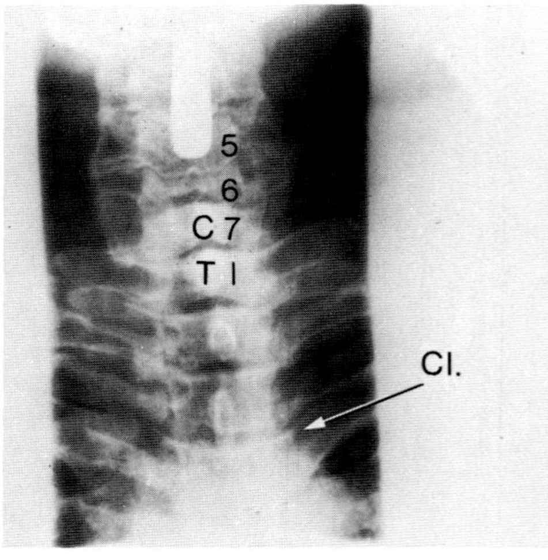


3 a

1
a

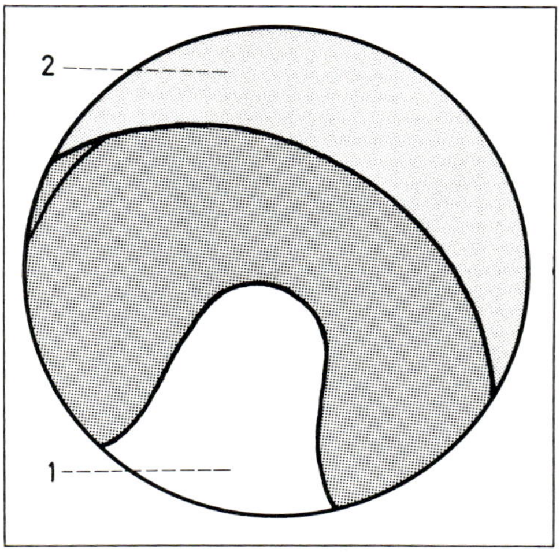


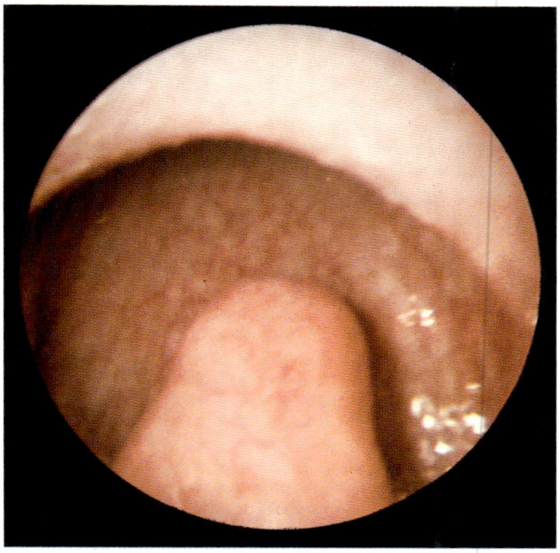

1
b

2
a

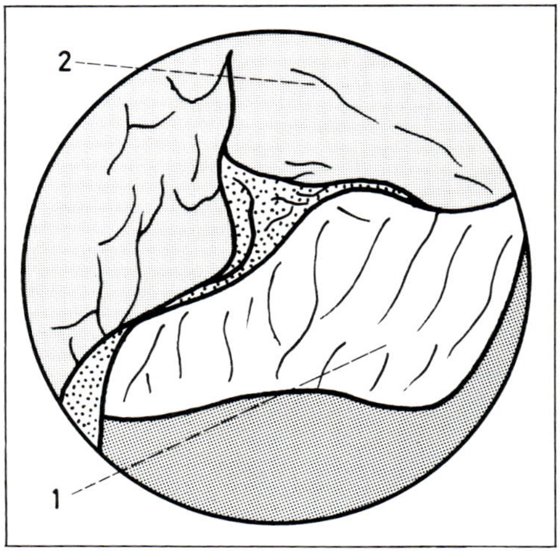


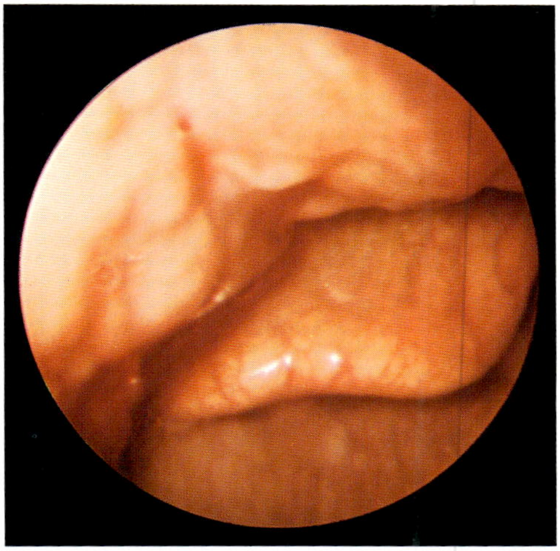

2
b

3
b

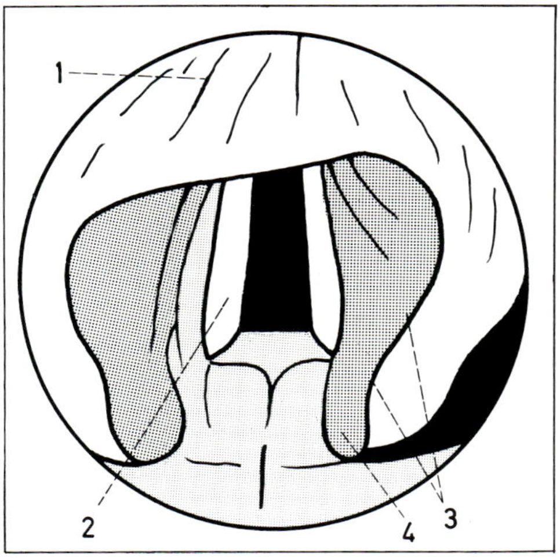


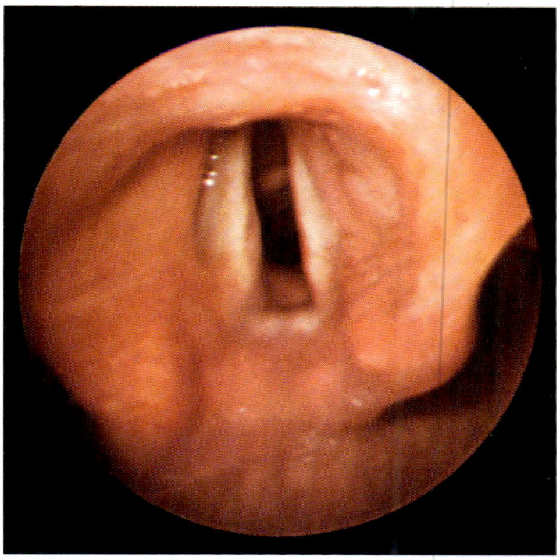

3
c

4 The vocal chords firmly closed during a gag maneuver. The aryepiglottic folds are prominent, especially the fold on the right which almost completely obscures the right vocal chord

5 Close-up view of tightly closed vocal chords. The bronchoscope should never be forced between closed vocal chords

6a, b The bevel of the bronchoscope is positioned vertically for insertion between the vocal chords. It is then advanced further while being rotated back to its initial horizontal position. *1* Bronchoscope; *2* left vocal chord

7a–c The bronchoscope positioned in the larynx just beyond the vocal chords. The cricoid cartilage is seen to describe a full circle. The level of the bronchoscope as shown in Fig. 7a is two full vertebrae lower than that depicted in Fig. 3a. *1* Cricoid cartilage; *2* tracheal cartilage

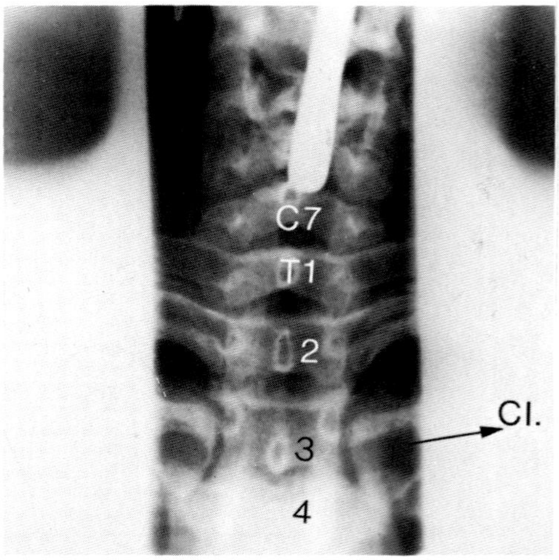


7
a

4

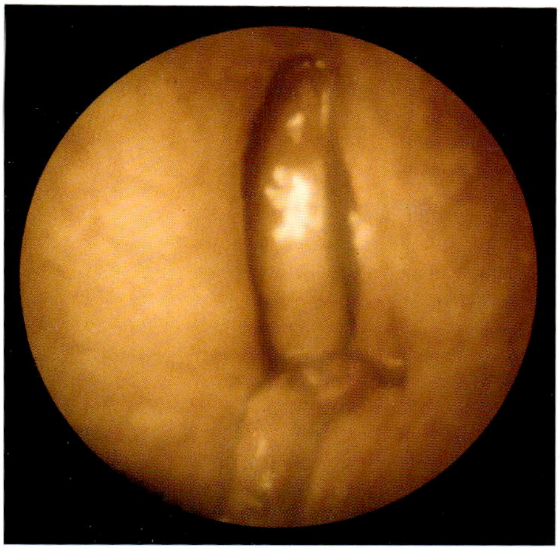

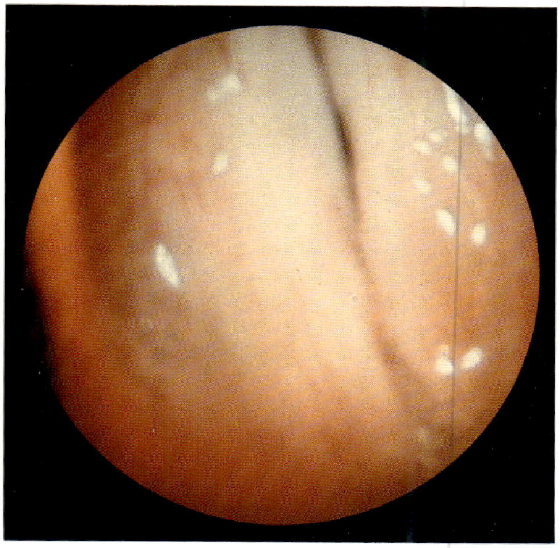

5

6
a

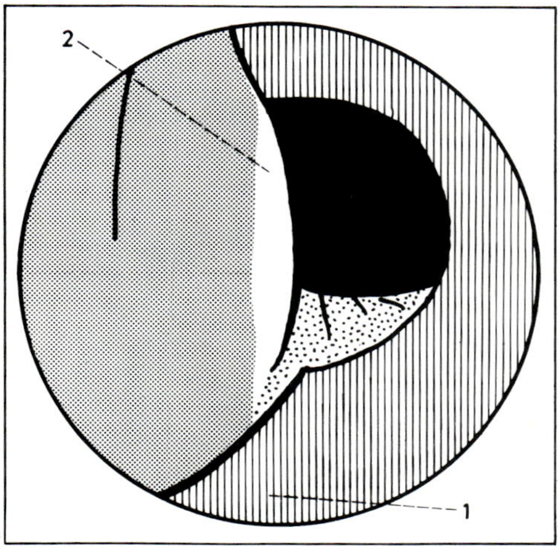


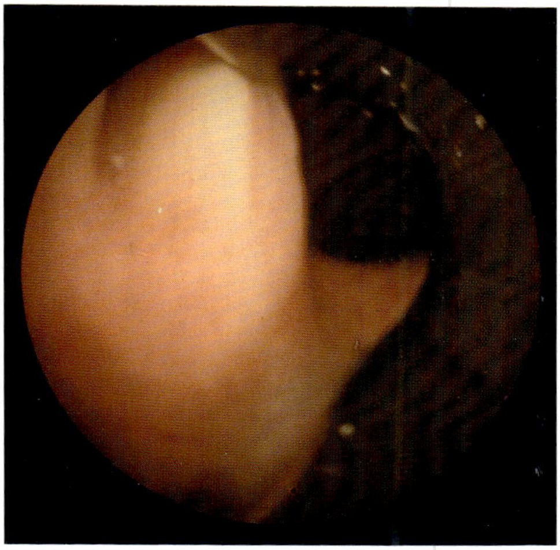

6
b

7
b

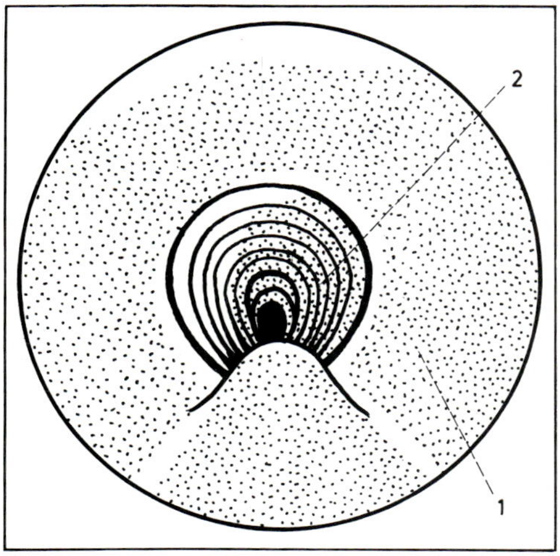


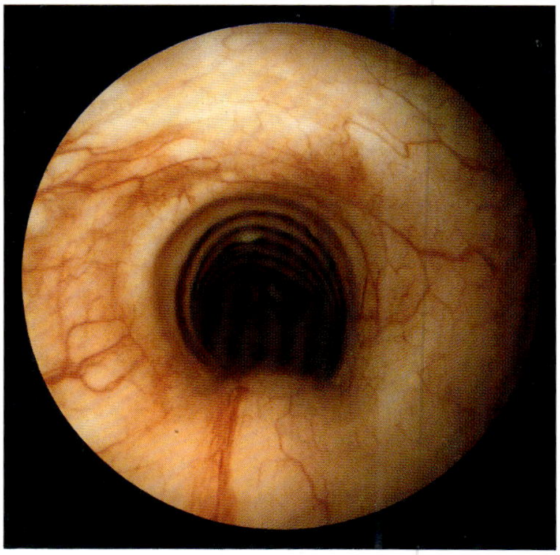

7
c

8 a–c The bronchoscope lodged in the extrathoracic portion of the trachea just distal to the cricoid cartilage. The level of the instrument in Fig. 8a is one vertebra below that shown in Fig. 7a. Note the C-shaped cartilage, which comprises a large segment of a circle, and the relatively narrow posterior membrane which occupies the minor segment. The paper-clip shown in Fig. 8a is at the level of the thoracic inlet. *1* Posterior membrane; *2* tracheal cartilage C-rings

9 a–c The bronchoscope here has been positioned at the level of the thoracic inlet, as can be seen from Fig. 9a, the paper-clip marker having been retained at this level. Note the broader posterior membrane according with the greater distance between the opposing ends of the cartilage. *1* Posterior membrane; *2* carina (tracheal bifurcation); *3* cartilage C-rings

10 a–c The bronchoscope positioned near the carina in the thoracic trachea. The broad posterior membrane is shown in relation to the distance between the ends of the C-shaped cartilages. With the head in this position the length of the intrathoracic trachea can be gauged from the space intervening between the paper-clip marker and the tip of the bronchoscope shown in Fig. 10a. *1* Carina; *2* right main bronchus; *3* left main bronchus; *4* posterior membrane

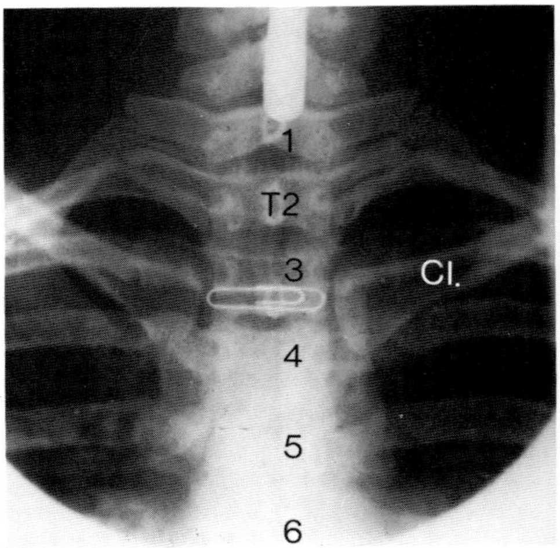


8
a

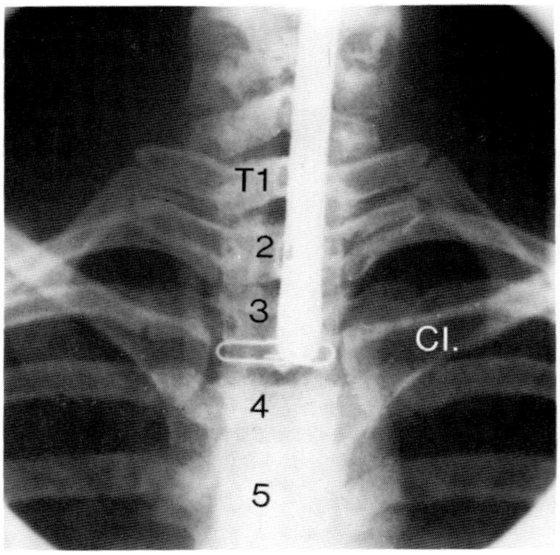


9
a

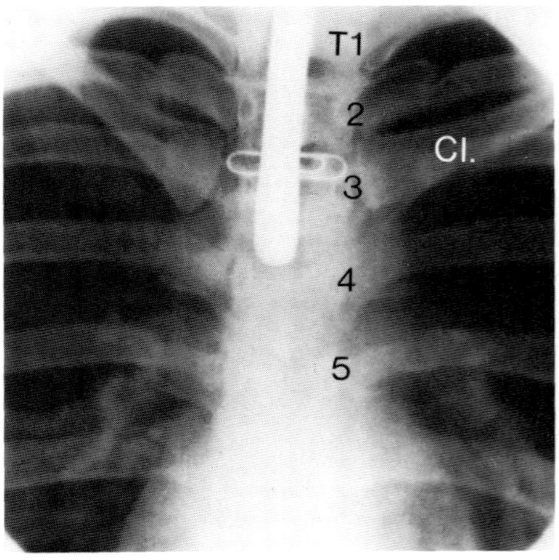


10
a

8
b

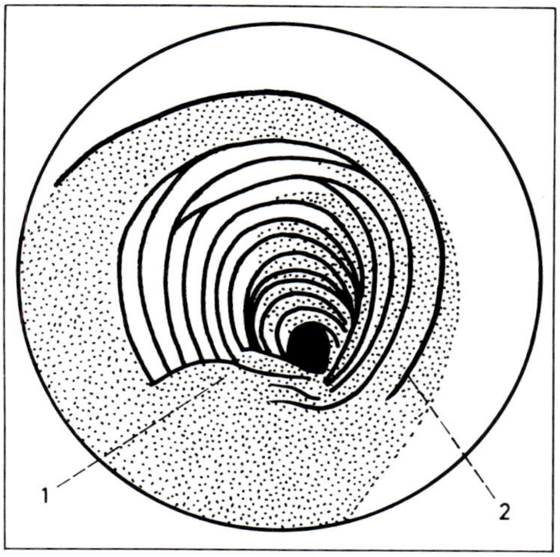


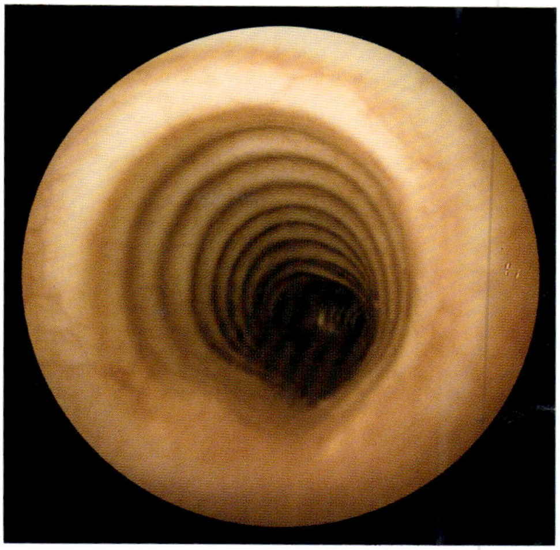

8
c

9
b

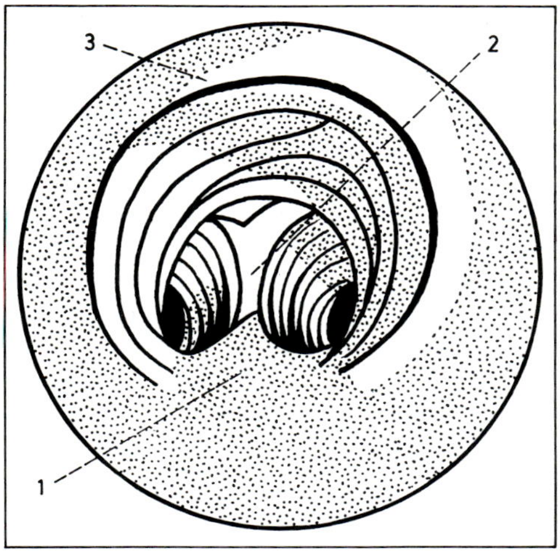


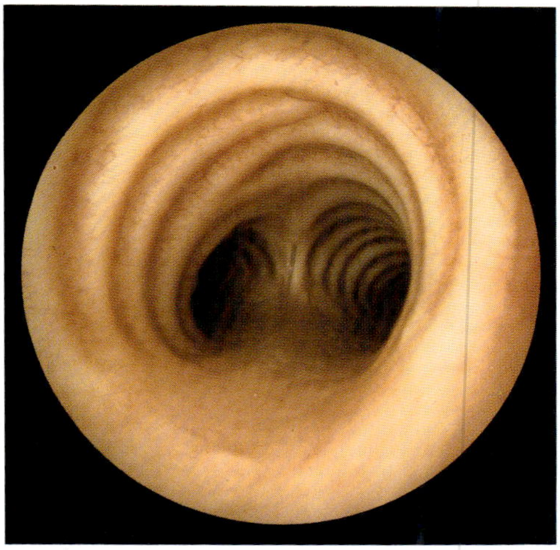

9
c

0
b

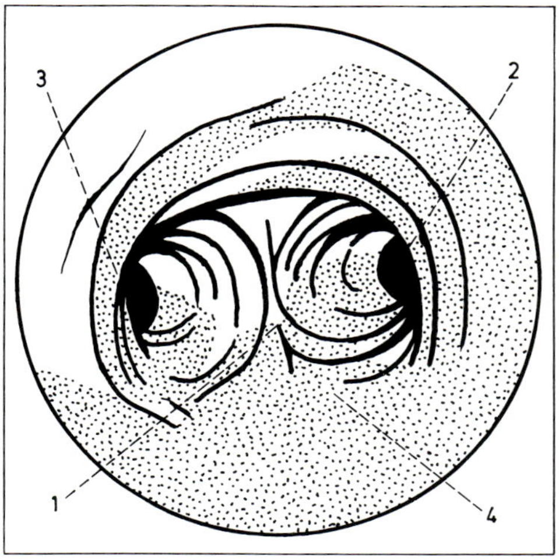


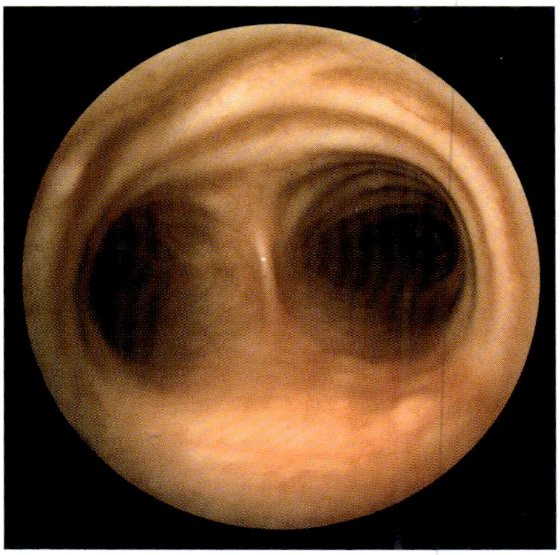

10
c

11 There is a sizeable variation in the width of the posterior membrane in individual subjects. Once again the bronchoscope has been positioned at the thoracic inlet, and the posterior membrane in this patient may be compared with the posterior membrane in Fig. 9

12 During forced expiration, the posterior membrane prolapses inward and tends to draw the opposing ends of the C-cartilages together to form an unbroken cartilaginous ring

13a, b The carina is sharp-edged and has relatively narrow bases on the anterior and posterior aspects. Note the distinct cartilaginous ring structure right up to the carina and also the mucosal corrugations on the posterior tracheal wall, dividing at the carina and continuing down the right and left main bronchi. *1* Carina; *2* cartilage of right bronchus forming a semicircle; *3* terminal tracheal cartilage; *4* mucosal corrugations

14 This demonstrates a normal sharp-edged carina during the inspiratory phase. It can assume a flattened and somewhat blunted appearance during expiration as illustrated by Fig. 15

15 The functionally changed appearance of the normal carina during the expiratory phase (cf. Fig. 14)

1

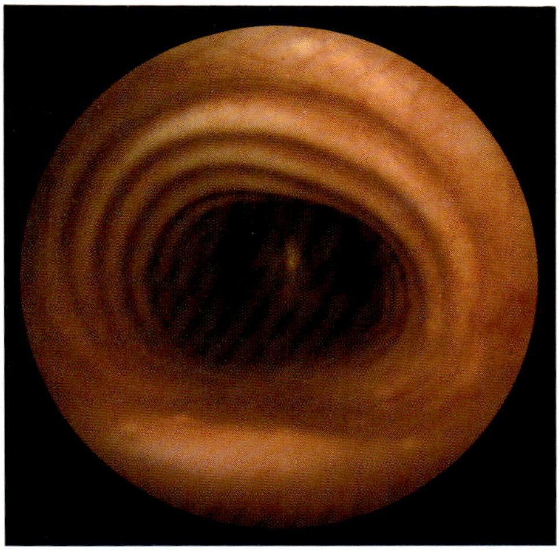

12

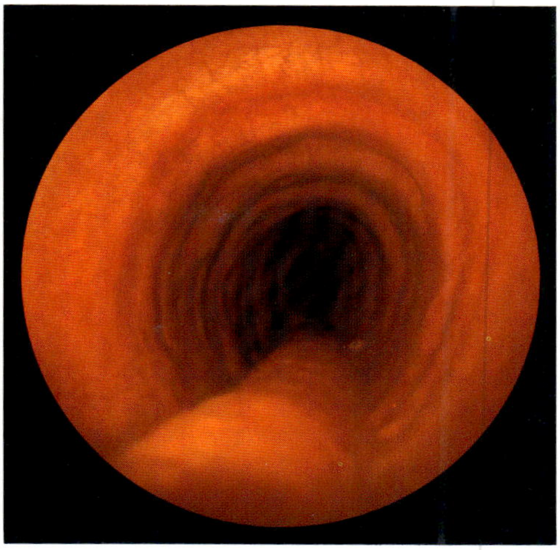

3
a

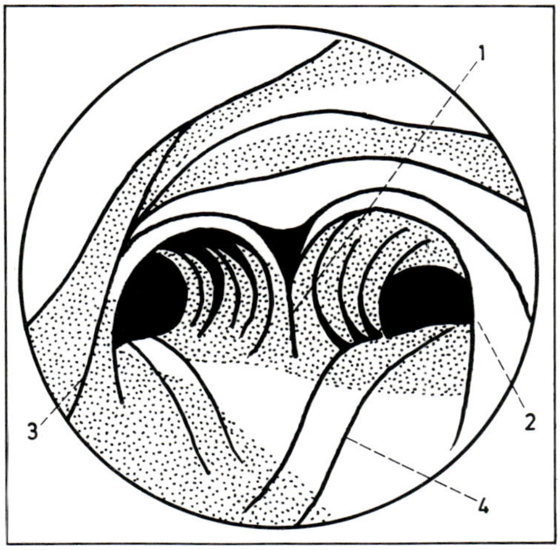


13
b

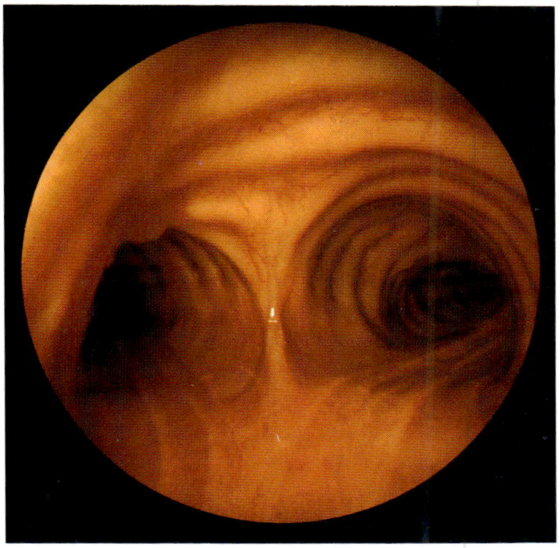

4

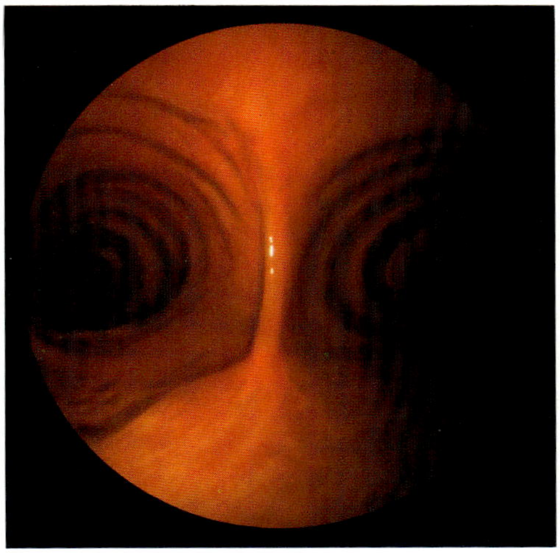

15

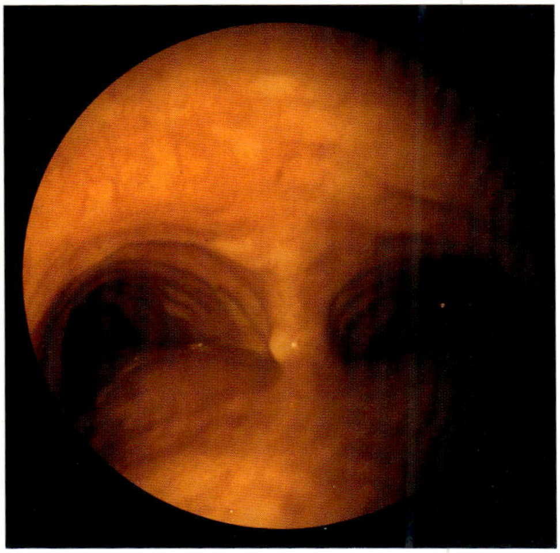

16a, b With the bronchoscope positioned just below the level of the carina, the right main bronchus can be seen, with the opening to the right upper lobe bronchus visible in the three o'clock position. Note the broad posterior membrane and the semicircular form of the bronchial cartilages. The mucosal corrugations are fairly prominent, and some of them are seen to branch off to the right where they enter the orifice of the right upper lobe bronchus. The level of the bronchoscope may be identified from Fig. 16a

17 a, b A view of the right upper lobe bronchus through the 30°-angled telescope. Note the mucosal corrugations branching off into the right upper lobe bronchus. Optical distortion through the 30°-angled telescope exaggerates the breadth of the bronchial spur. This appearance should not be confused with a pathologically broadened spur, which may also be distinguished by its immobility. *1* Right main bronchus; *2* opening to right upper lobe bronchus; *3* mucosal corrugations

18a, b A view of the right upper lobe bronchus through the 90°-angled telescope. The anterior segmental orifice is in the one o'clock position, the posterolateral orifice at nine o'clock, and the apical orifice at five o'clock. *1* Anterior orifice; *2* posterior orifice; *3* apical orifice; *4* mucosal corrugation

16 a

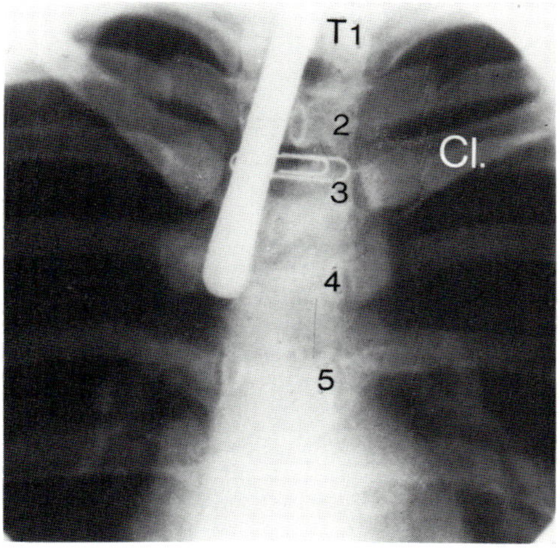


16 b

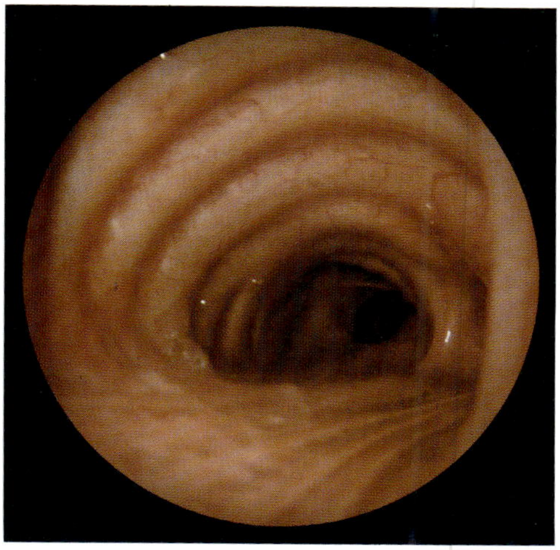

17 a

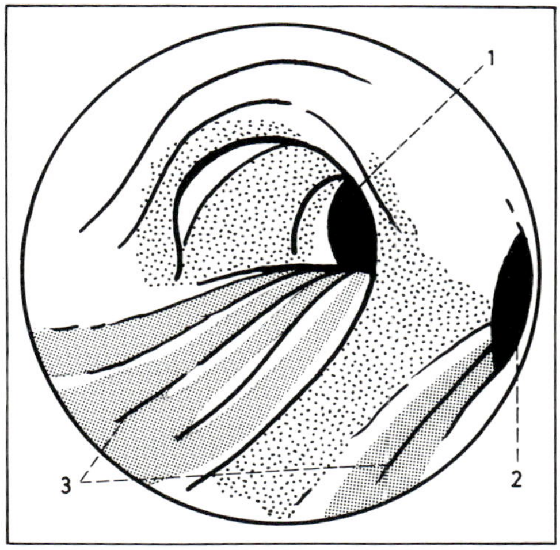


17 b

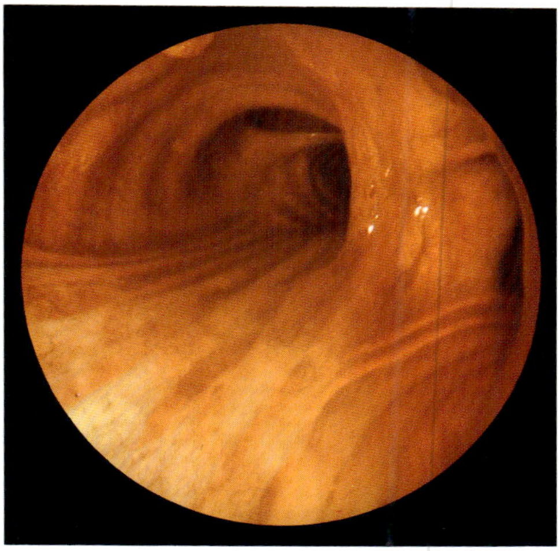

18 a

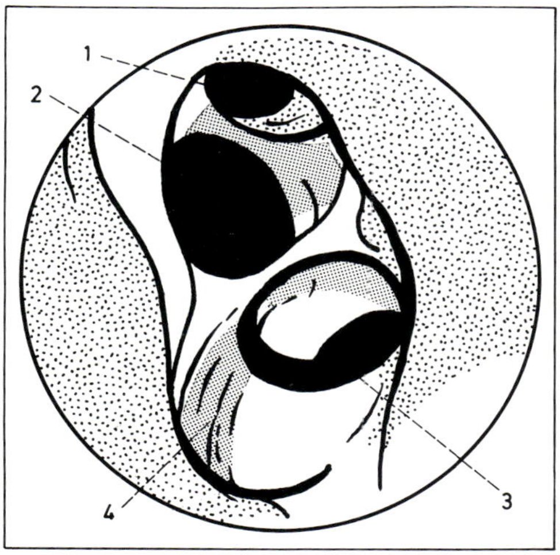


18 b

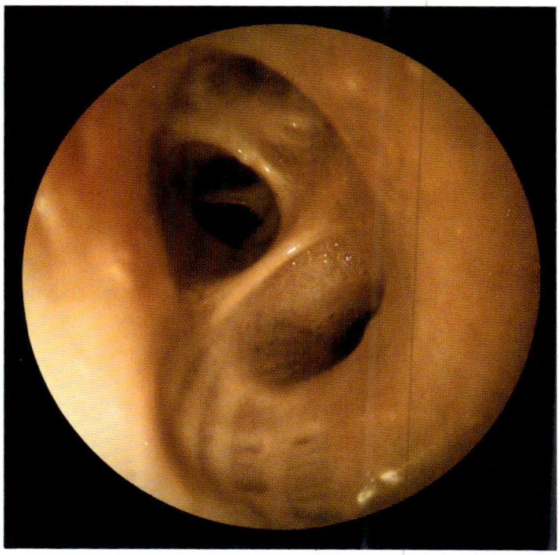

19 a, b The bronchoscope positioned just beyond the level of the right upper lobe bronchial opening, affording a view down the intermediate bronchus, with the right middle lobar orifice visible at twelve o'clock and the opening to the apical segment of the right lower lobe to be seen distally. Note the prominent mucosal corrugations. The level of the bronchoscope can be seen in Fig. 19 a

20 a–c The bronchoscope positioned at the end of the intermediate bronchus with the middle lobe opening at twelve o'clock, the opening to the apical segment of the lower lobe at six o'clock, and the basal segmental orifices viewed distally. The level of the bronchoscope is shown in Fig. 20 a. *1* Middle lobe bronchus; *2* basal segments of lower lobe; *3* apical segment of lower lobe; *4* mucosal corrugations; *5* spur of middle lobe bronchus

20 a

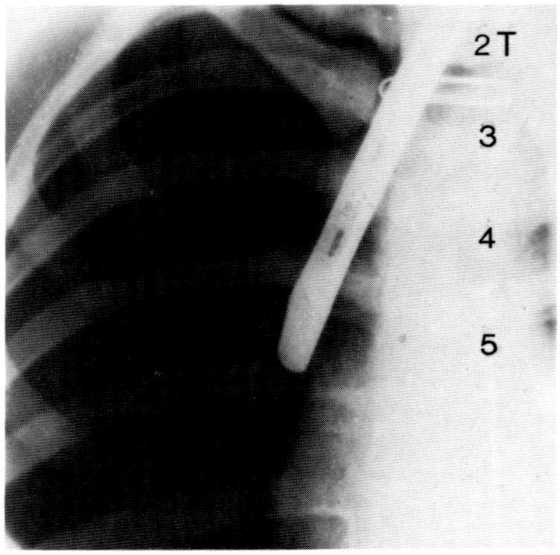


21 a–c With the tip of the bronchoscope at the level of the middle lobe bronchus, a portion of the opening to the apical segment of the lower lobe can be seen in the five o'clock position. The medial basal segmental orifice is at nine o'clock, and the remaining basal segmental openings are glimpsed more distally. The level of the bronchoscope is shown in Fig. 21 a. *1* Part of the opening to apical segment of the lower lobe; *2* openings of enlarged submucosal glands as seen in chronic bronchitis; *3* anterolateral basal segmental bronchus; *4* medial basal segmental bronchus; *5* posterior basal segmental bronchus

21 a

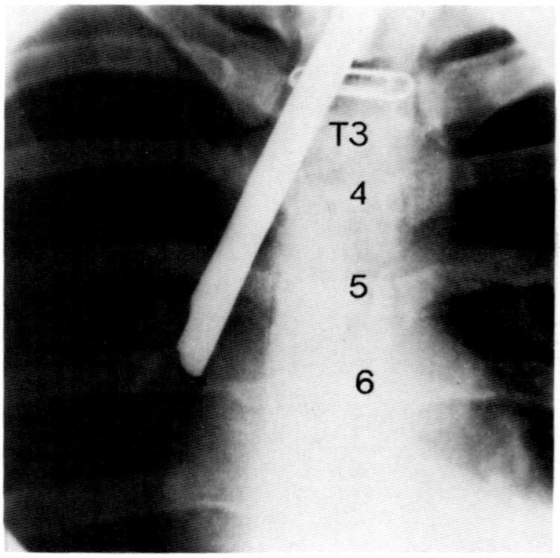

9
a

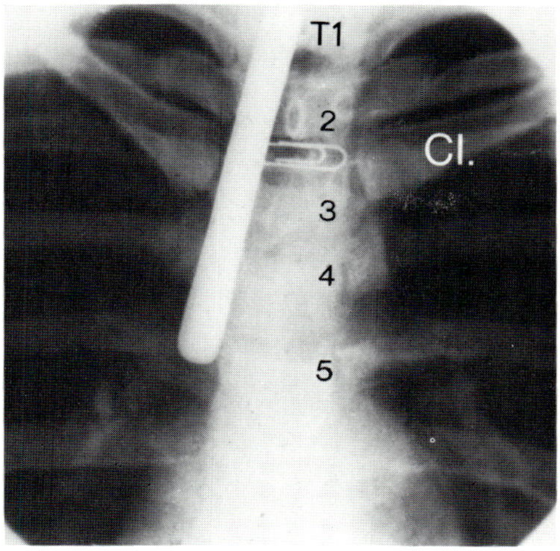


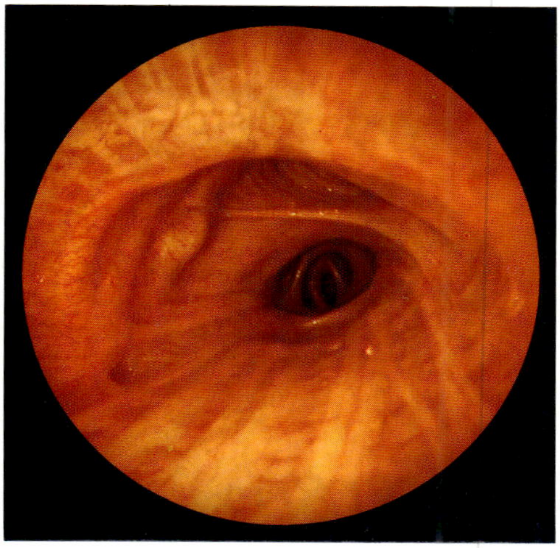

19
b

20
b

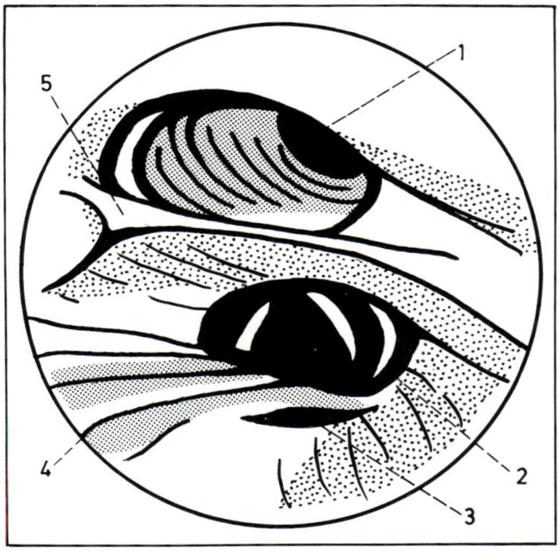


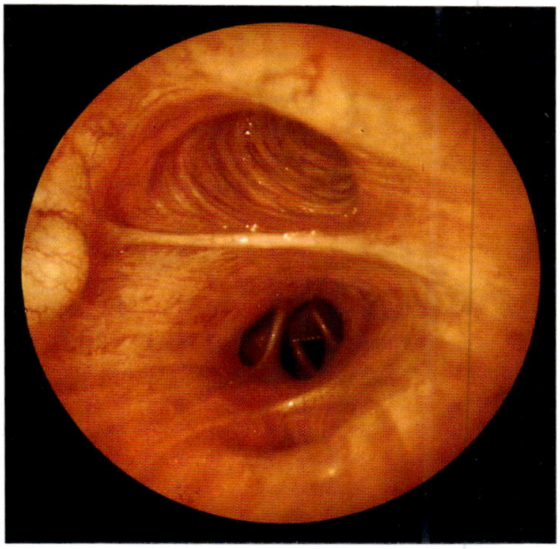

20
c

21
b

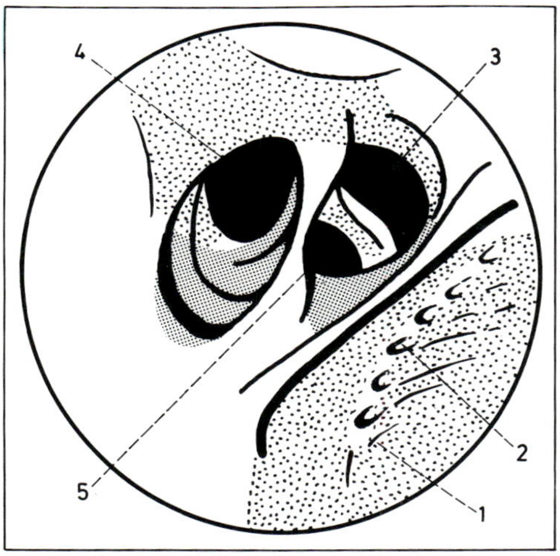


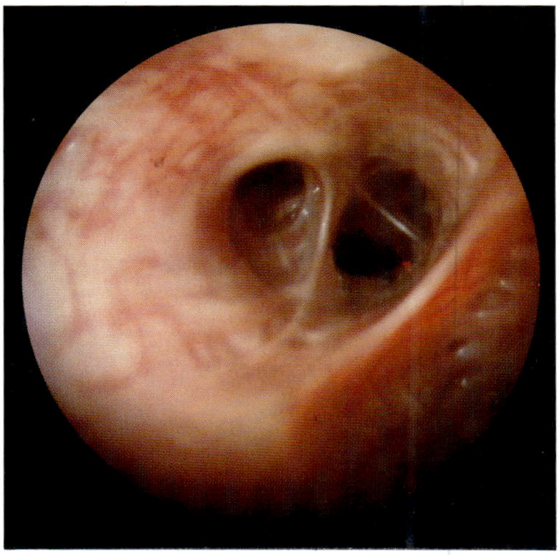

21
c

22a, b With the tip of the bronchoscope at the carina and with the patient's head rotated slightly to the right, the left main bronchus is visualized. The level of the bronchoscope is shown in Fig. 22a

23a, b With the bronchoscope in position in the left main bronchus, the leftward curvature of this bronchus can be seen, and it will be appreciated that the tip of the bronchoscope will impinge on the medial wall as it is advanced down the left main bronchus. Note the prominent mucosal corrugations on the posterior membrane. The level of the bronchoscope is demonstrated in Fig. 23a

24a–c The spur of the left upper lobe bronchial orifice is sharp and forms a virtual second carina. The left upper lobe bronchial orifice appears in the ten o'clock position, while the opening to the apical segment of the lower lobe is seen just slightly lower down at six o'clock. The level of the bronchoscope can be gauged from Fig. 24a. *1* Opening to left upper lobe; *2* left lower lobe bronchus; *3* lower lobe apical segmental opening

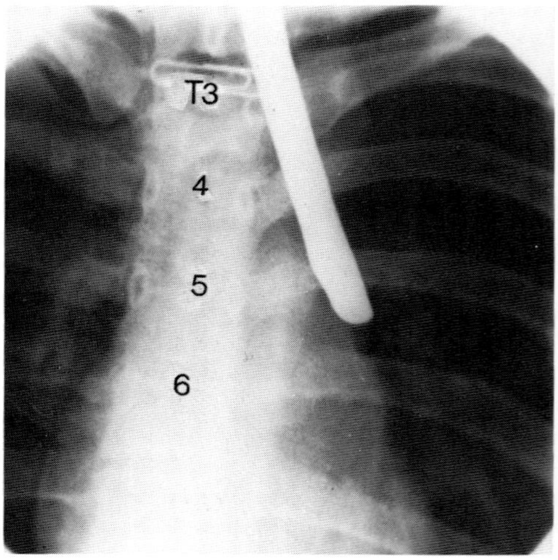


24 a

22
a

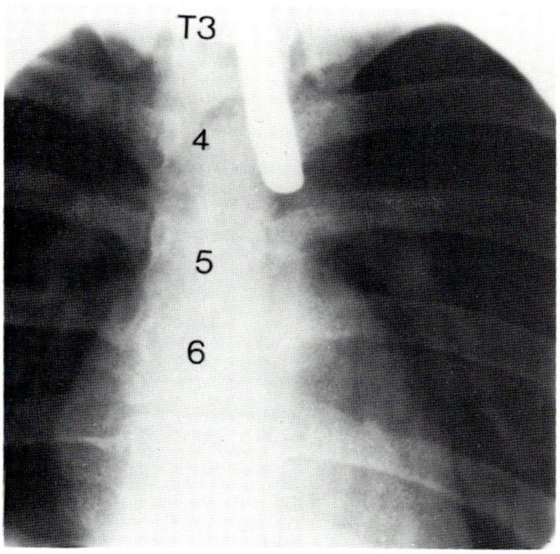


22
b

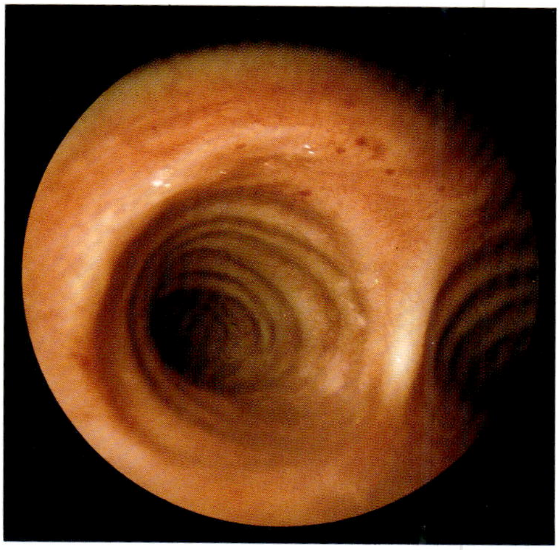

23
a

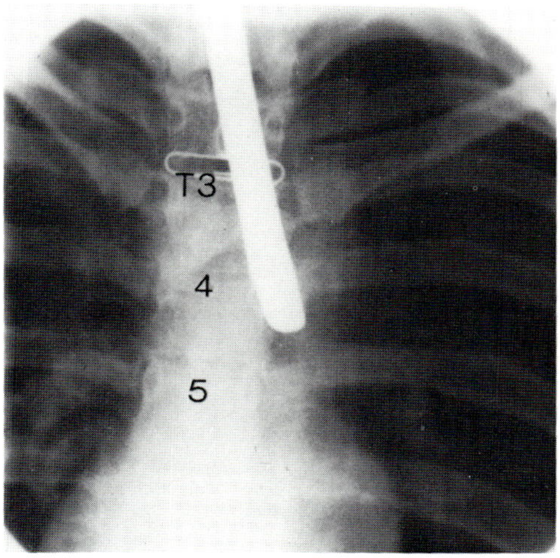


23
b

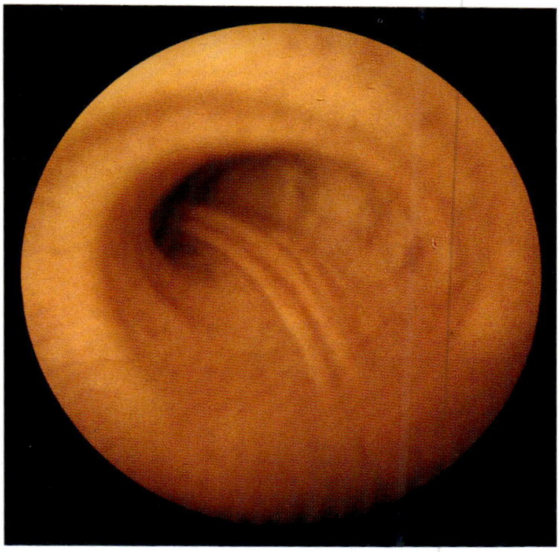

24
b

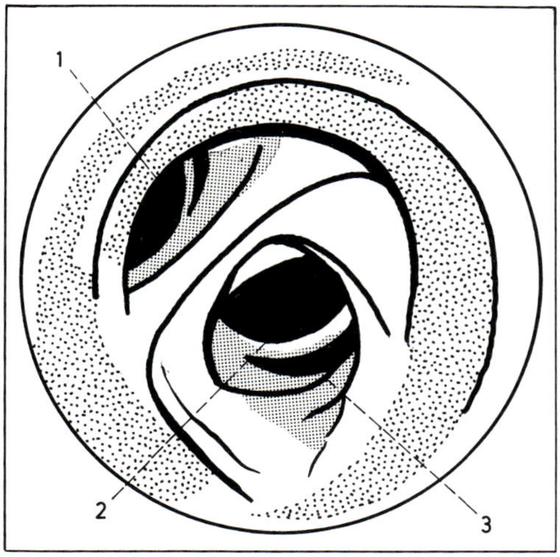


24
c

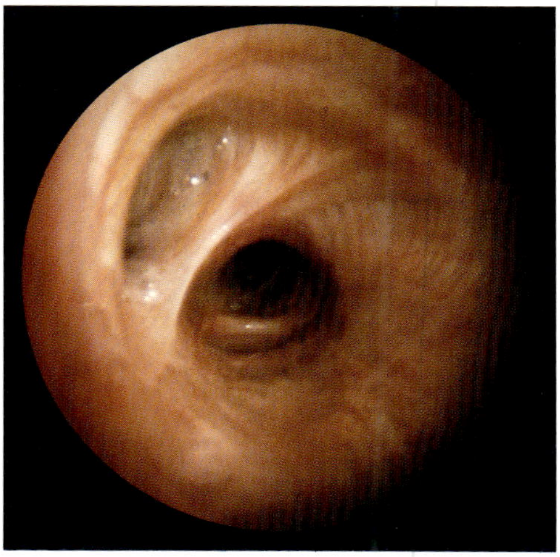

25a, b With a 30°-angled telescope the left upper lobe bronchial opening is clearly visualized on the left, while the bronchus supplying the lingula originates from the left upper lobe bronchus in the two o'clock position. *1* Lingular segmental orifice; *2* upper division segmental orifice; *3* lower basal bronchi; *4* opening to apical segment of lower lobe

26a, b Occasionally, as shown in this view, the lingular bronchus arises much nearer the left main bronchus. Its orifice is, however, still seen to lie immediately to the left of the left upper lobe bronchial spur but somewhat to the right of the left anterior and apical segmental openings. *1* Lower lobe bronchus; *2* opening to lingular bronchus; *3* opening to anterior and apical segmental bronchi

27a, b With the 30°-angled telescope positioned at the level of the left upper lobe bronchial spur, the lower lobe apical segmental orifice is clearly visualized, with the basal bronchi seen distally. *1* Left upper lobe bronchial opening; *2* left upper lobe bronchial spur; *3* lower lobe bronchial orifice; *4* opening to apical segmental bronchus

25 a

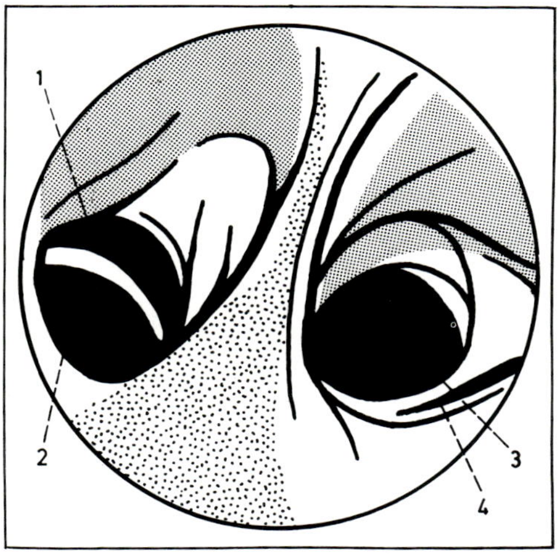


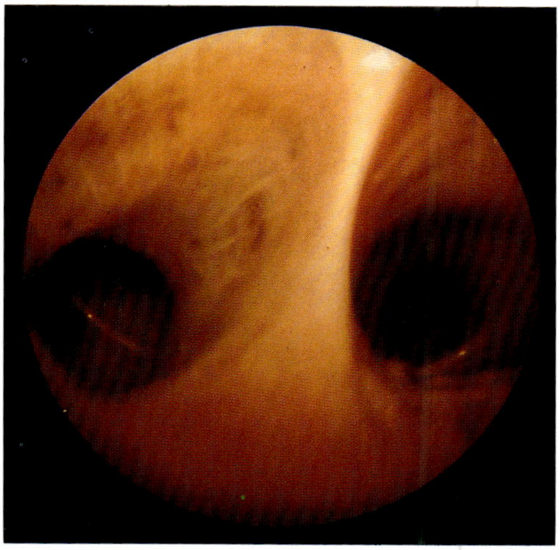

25 b

26 a

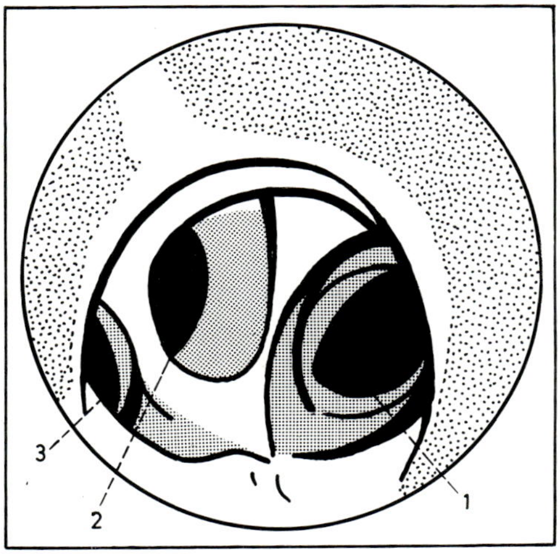


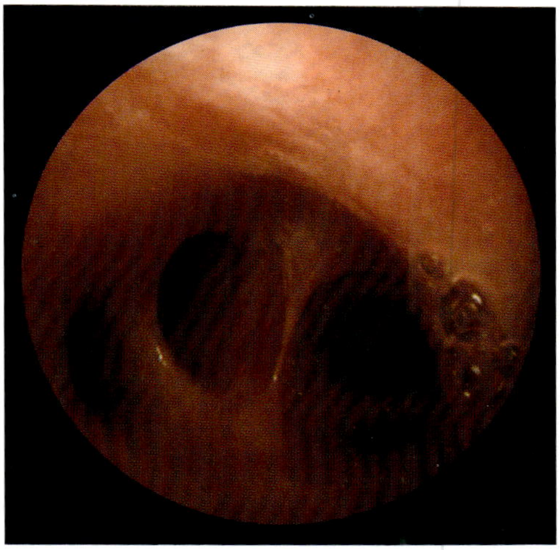

26 b

27 a

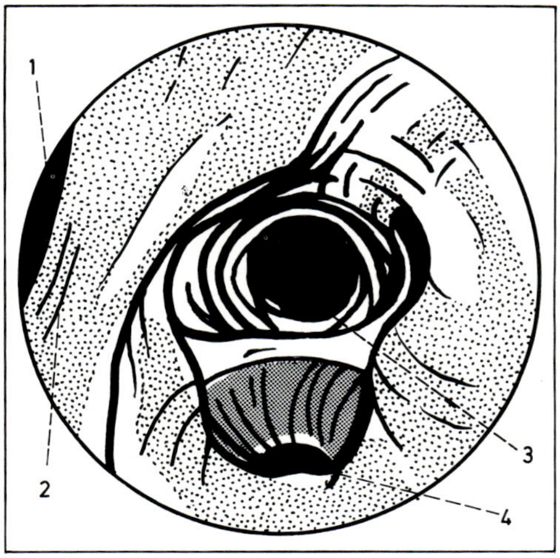


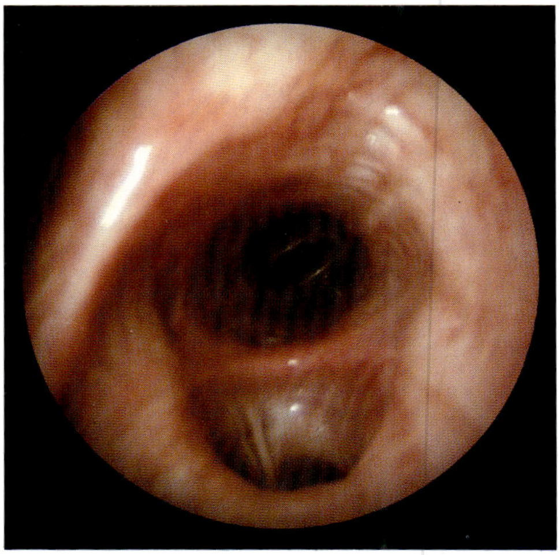

27 b

28a, b Positioning the telescope distally to the apical segmental orifice, the rim of which can just be seen at five o'clock, brings the basal segmental openings into view. This plate illustrates a common anatomical variation, namely a bifurcation of the lower lobe bronchus (see text). *1* Opening to anterior and medial segments; *2* opening to lateral and posterior segments

*Dynamic Changes in the Bronchial Tree Under Conditions of Quiet Respiration or Coughing*

29 The vocal chords during inspiration

30 The vocal chords during expiration

31 When the tracheal cartilages of different patients as seen through a bronchoscope positioned at the level of the thoracic inlet are compared, great structural variation in the cartilage is observed. In this view, the cartilage comprises a large segment of the tracheal circle, and the posterior membrane is narrow

32 In comparison with Fig. 31, the tracheal cartilages comprise a smaller segment of the full circle, and the posterior membrane is consequently broader

28 a

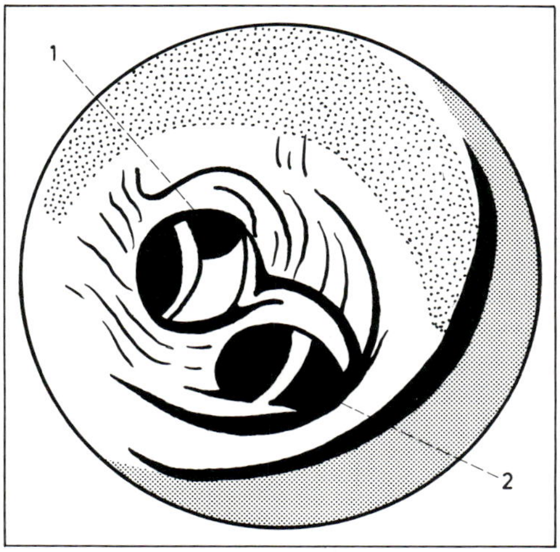


28 b

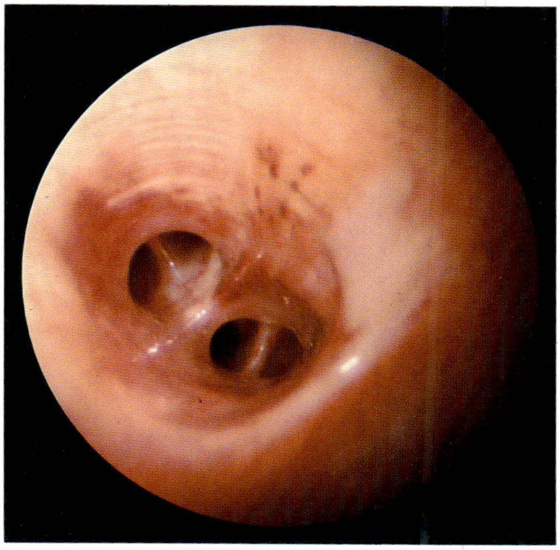

29

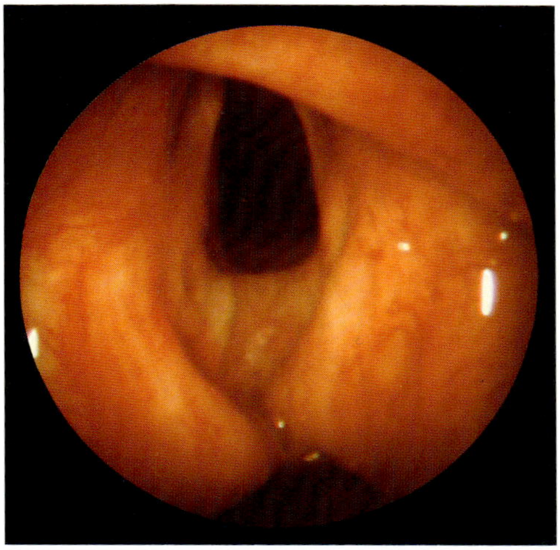

30

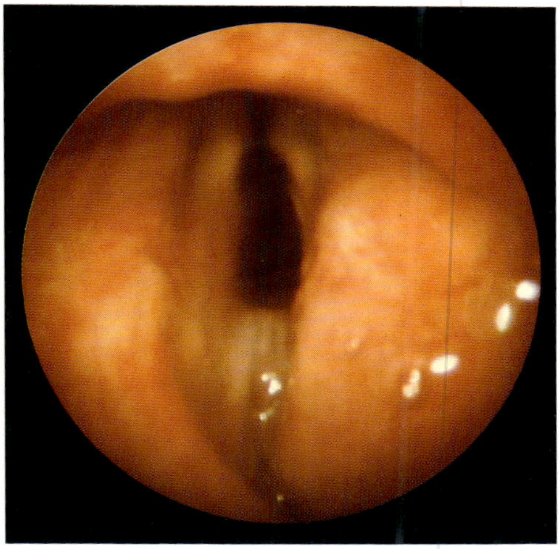

31

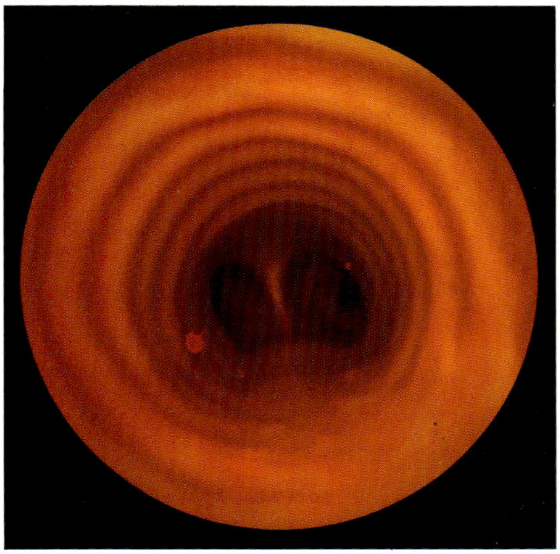

32

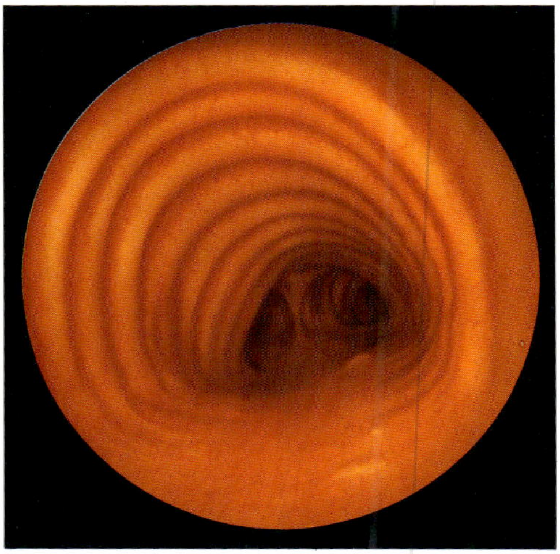

33 In contrast to the appearances in the patients illustrated in Figs. 31 and 32, this view, obtained at a comparable level in the trachea, displays semicircular cartilage form

34 Viewing the trachea lower down towards the carina, a comparison with Figs. 31–33 reveals that the cartilages may comprise even smaller segments of the full circle, the posterior membrane being proportionately broader

35 Inward bulging of the posterior membrane at the level of the carina and the two main bronchi occurs even during normal quiet expiration. Note the broad posterior membrane and semicircular cartilaginous structure of the two main bronchi

36 There is a posterior excursion of the posterior membrane during the inspiratory phase, so that membrane and cartilages together describe a complete circle

37 During a forced expiratory maneuver or cough, the posterior membrane prolapses into the tracheal lumen, and by its traction tends to approximate the ends of the cartilages so that the latter themselves complete the ring structure. This inward bulge is more pronounced in the presence of bronchospasm (see text)

38 The lesser degree of posterior membrane prolapse apparent when this view is compared with that in Fig. 37 illustrates in the same patient the effect of administering bronchodilators (see text)

33

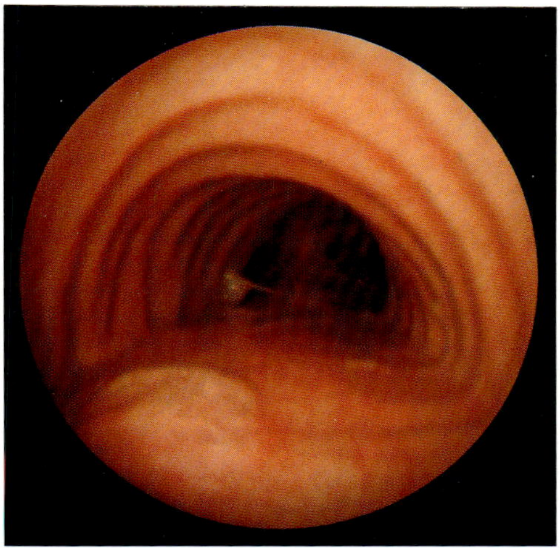

34

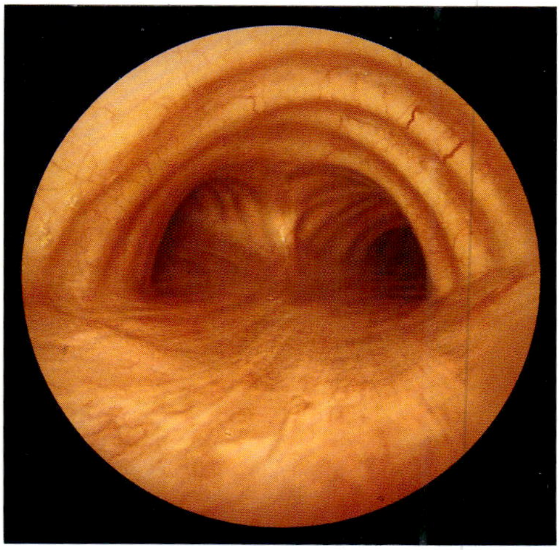

35

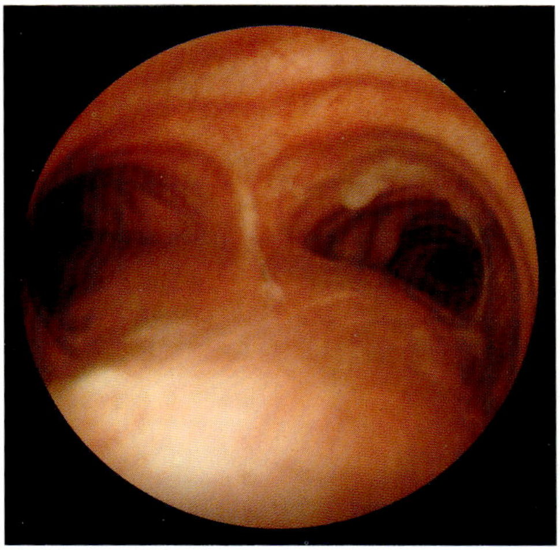

36

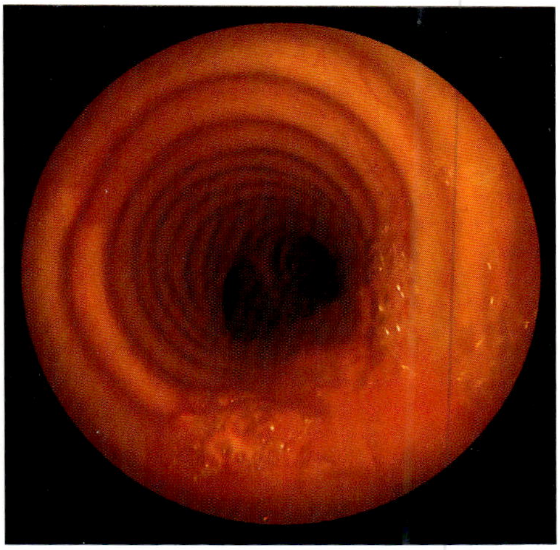

37

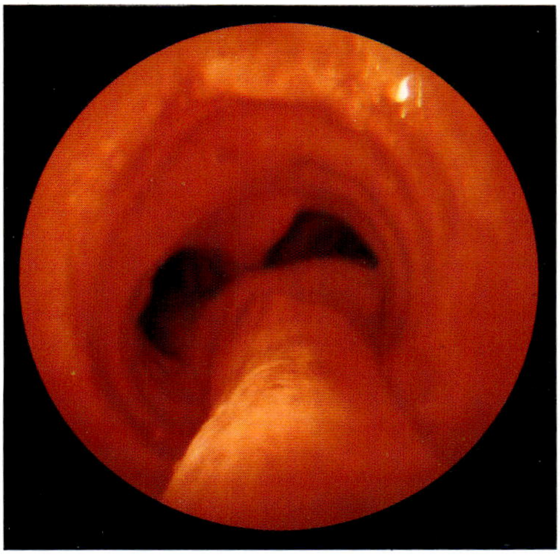

38

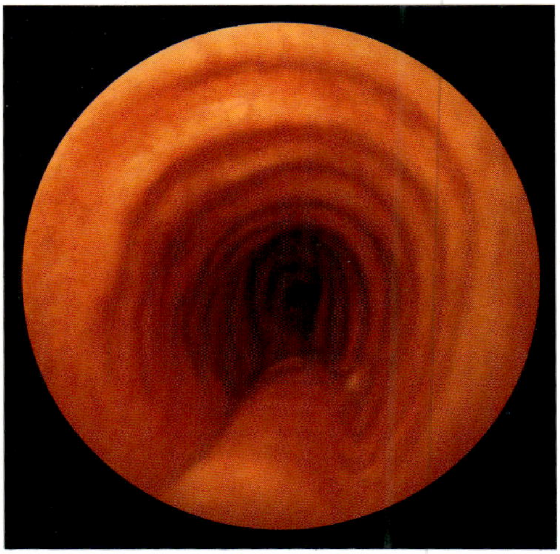

39 When this illustration is compared with Fig. 37, it is clear that the intraluminal prolapse of the posterior membrane is greatly accentuated where a trachea has cartilages of semicircular form and the membrane is broad. The indrawing of the ends of the cartilaginous ring structure to form a complete circle is not possible in such instances

40 Note the broad posterior membrane of the right main bronchus and the mucosal corrugations on this membrane. The posterior excursion of the membrane during inspiration does not result in the formation of a complete circle as is the case in the trachea

41 During forced expiratory maneuvers, the posterior membrane prolapses into the lumen of the right main bronchus, resulting in relatively greater encroachment on the lumen than is seen in the trachea. Note the mucosal corrugation which may here be of significance in promoting laminar air flow

42 Note the sagging of the anterior wall of the cartilaginous ring structure, as seen in a patient with chronic persistent cough. This deformity is more likely to occur in patients with a broad posterior membrane

43a, b The straightening and flattening of the right lateral wall of the trachea in a patient with chronic bronchitis. *1* Left main bronchus; *2* right main bronchus; *3* straightening of right lateral wall

39

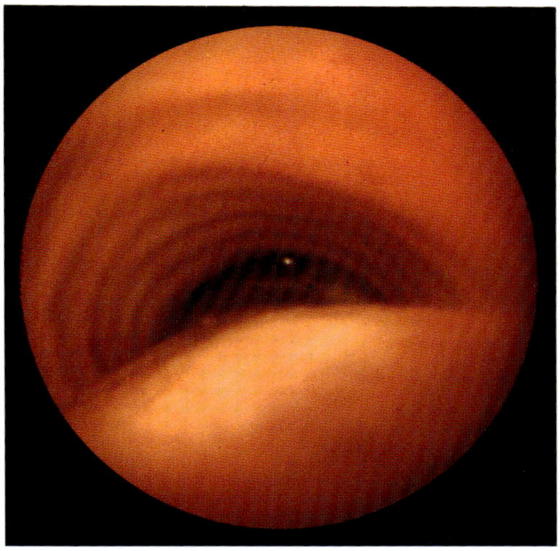

40

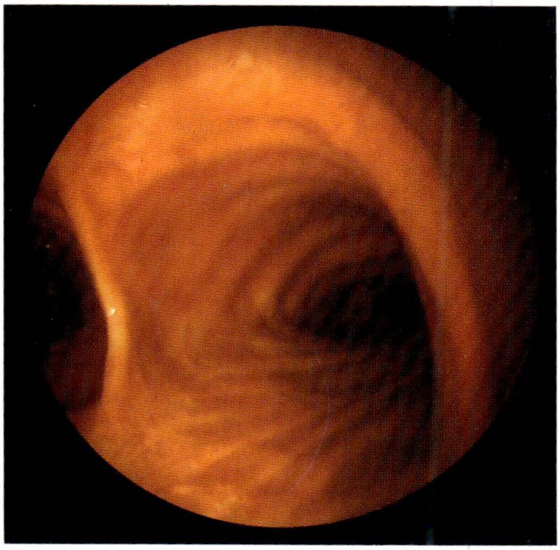

41

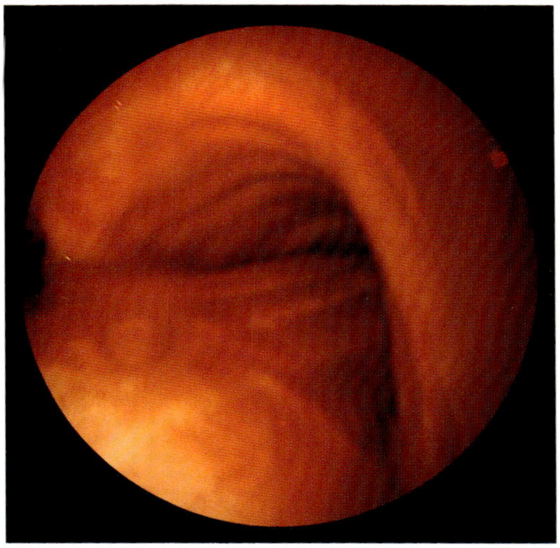

42

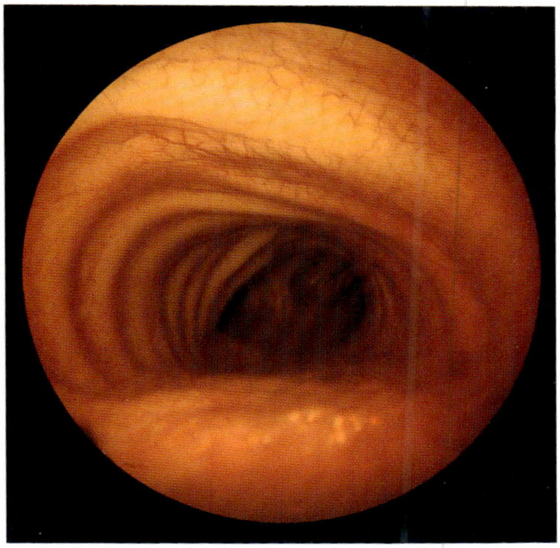

43 a

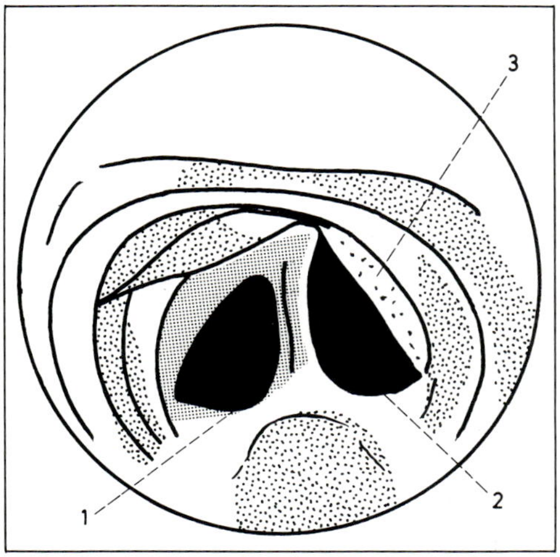


43 b

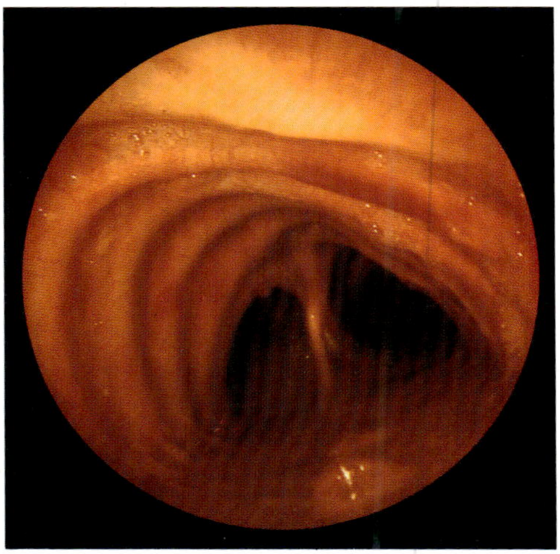

44a, b For comparison with Fig. 43, the straightening of the left lateral wall of the trachea in a patient with chronic bronchitis is shown in this view. *1* Left main bronchus; *2* right main bronchus; *3* straightening of left lateral wall

45 In a chronic bronchitic patient following a prolonged period of coughing, bilateral straightening and flattening of the walls as illustrated in Figs. 43 and 44 may develop to form a triangular trachea. Note the thickening at the apex, which is probably caused by the hinging effect produced when the posterior membrane prolapses into the lumen and approximates the opposing ends of the cartilage (see text)

46 Here, in the same patient as in Fig. 45, an expiratory maneuver results in total occlusion of the tracheal lumen

47a, b U-shaped tracheal cartilages. This deformity is not due to lateral pressure on the trachea but rather to the inability of the trachea to shorten during expiration (see text). *1* Posterior membrane; *2* U-shaped cartilage

44 a

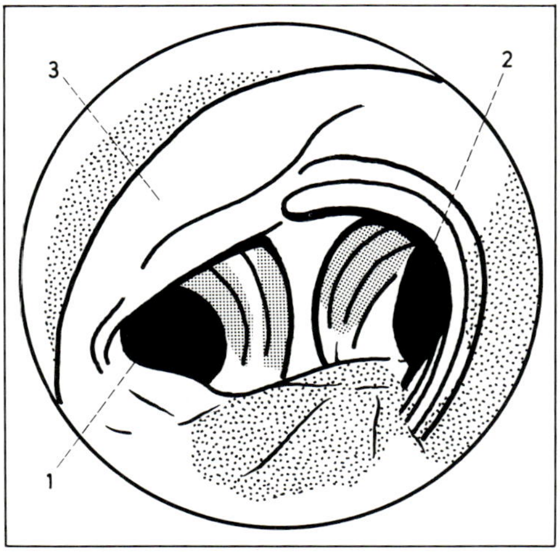


44 b

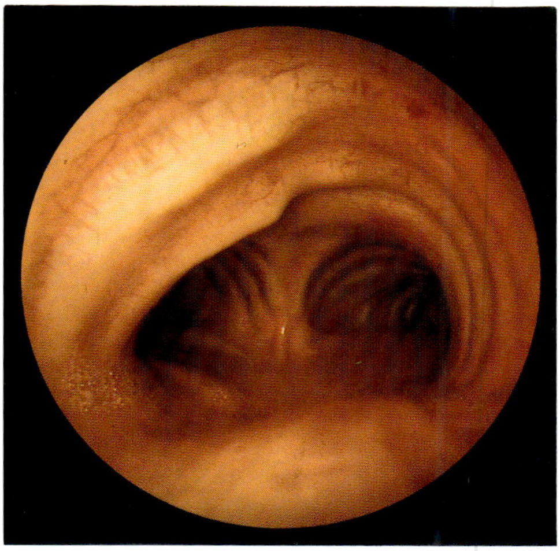

45

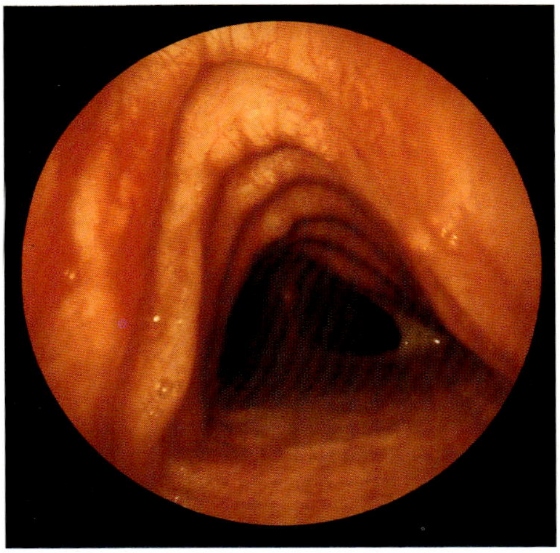

46

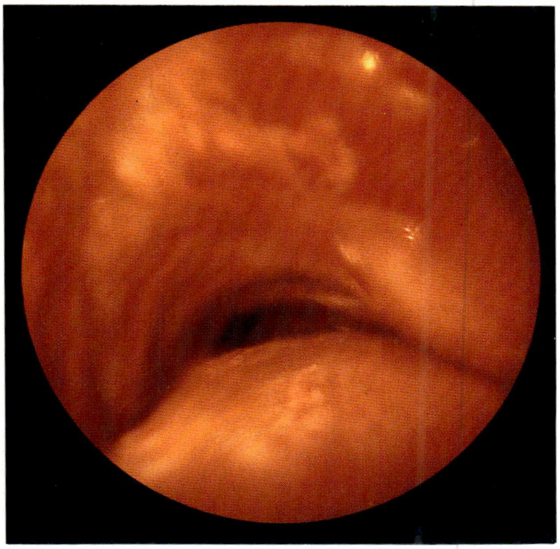

47 a

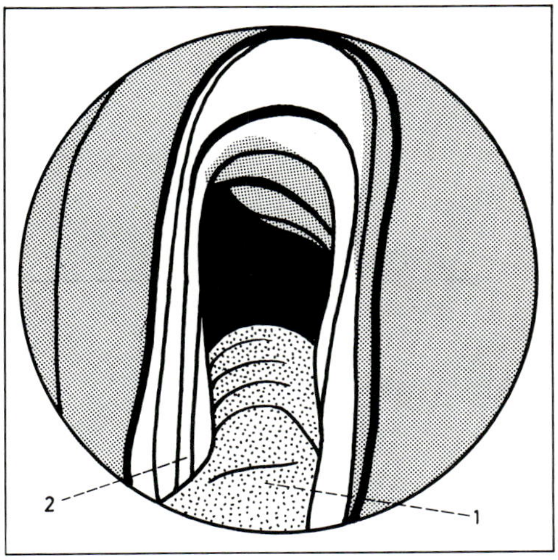


47 b

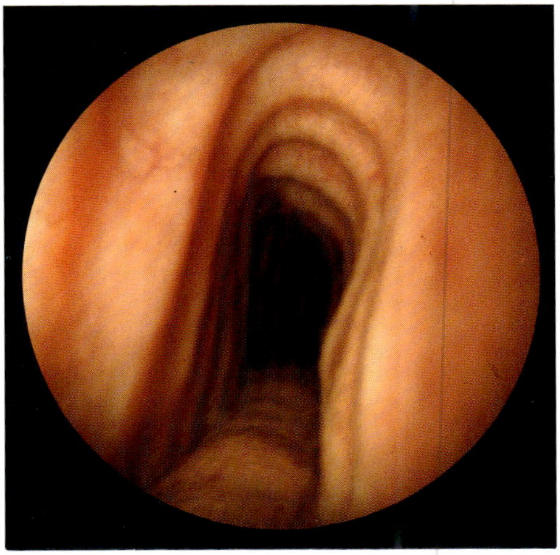

48 The side-to-side occlusion of the tracheal lumen due to kinking

49 The same patient as in Fig. 48, showing a side-to-side narrowing of the trachea at the level of the carina, also involving the main bronchi. Note also the prolapse of the posterior membrane at this level, drawing the lateral walls of the cartilage closer together, further diminishing the lumen of the trachea and main bronchi

50 The right main bronchus during inspiration in a patient with chronic bronchitis. Note the enlarged submucosal gland opening in the seven o'clock position. This is a common finding in chronic bronchitis

51 Same patient as in Fig. 50 during expiratory phase of cough. Note total distortion of bronchus, with total occlusion of lower lobe bronchus

52a, b Distortion of the left lower lobe bronchus at the commencement of an expiratory maneuver is shown here, the patency of the left upper lobe bronchial opening being maintained. *1* Opening to left upper lobe bronchus; *2* partially obstructed opening to left lower lobe bronchus; *3* mucosal corrugations

48

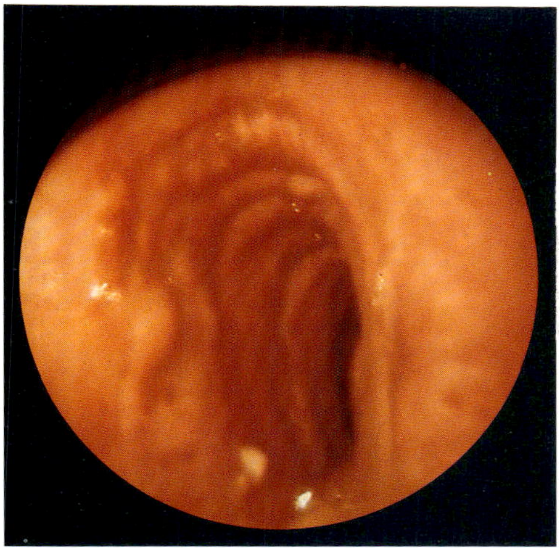

49

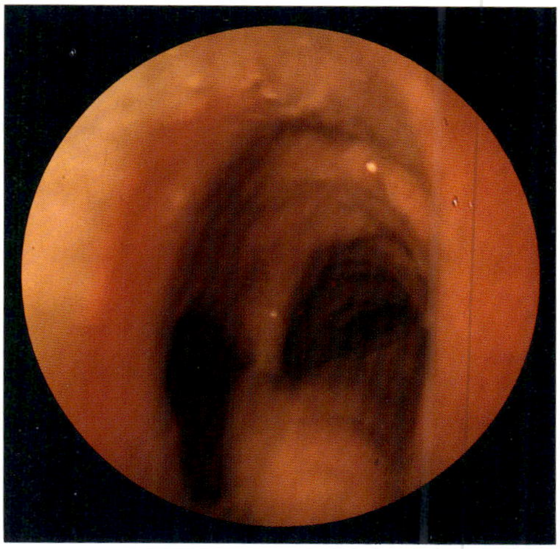

50

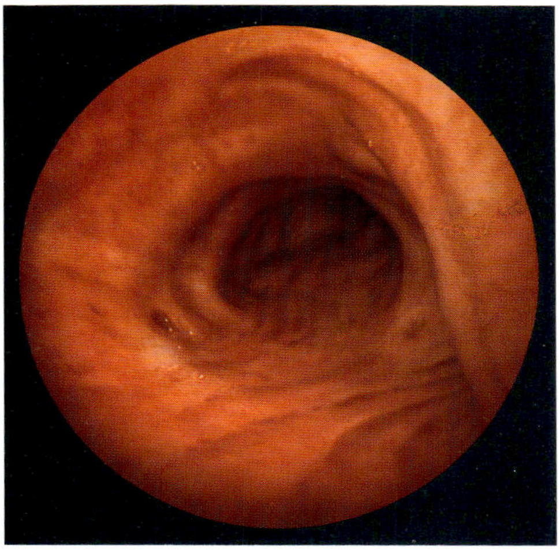

51

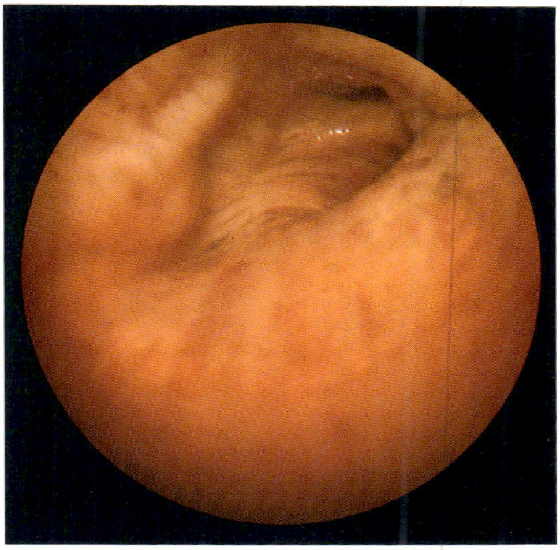

52
a

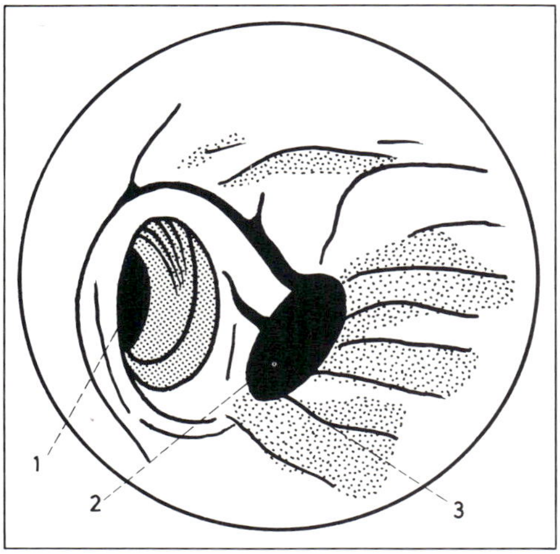


52
b

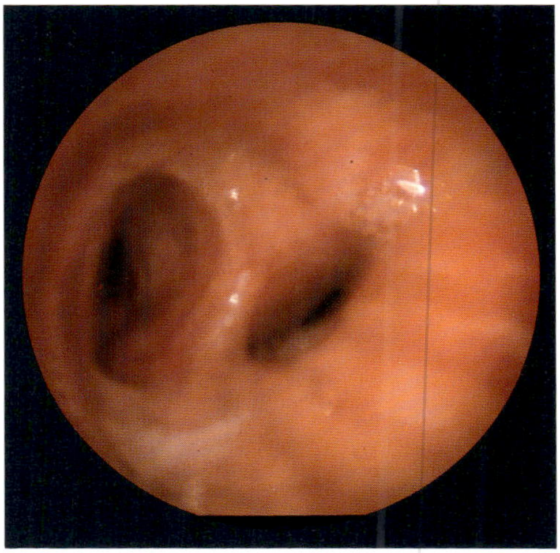

53a, b The same patient as in Fig. 52, showing almost total occlusion of the left lower lobe bronchial lumen. *1* Opening to left upper lobe bronchus; *2* totally obstructed opening to left lower lobe bronchus; *3* mucosal corrugations

54 The bronchoscope positioned at the level of the right middle lobe bronchial orifice

55 Bronchial spasm occurring after mechanical stimulation. Note the narrowed middle lobe opening and the droplets of clear mucus

56 Reactive hyperemia following mechanical stimulation in a chronic bronchitic patient

*Tumors*

57 Benign cyst of the epiglottis

53 a

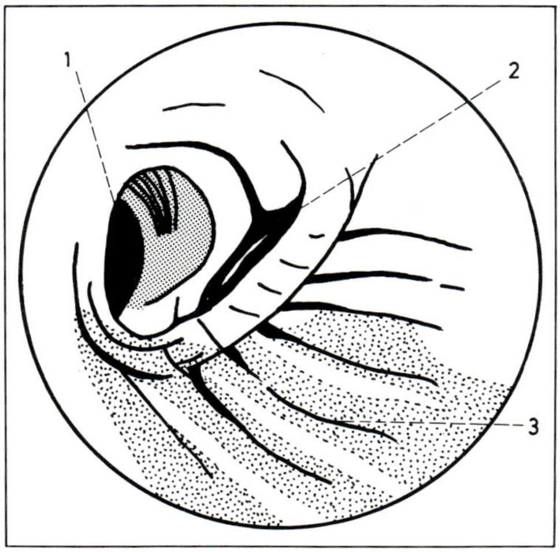


53 b

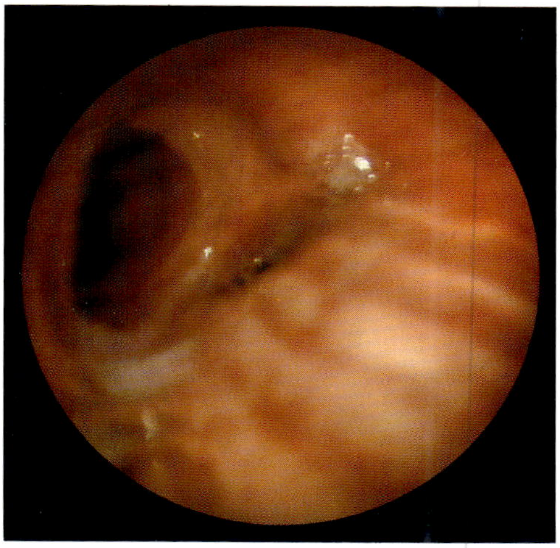

54

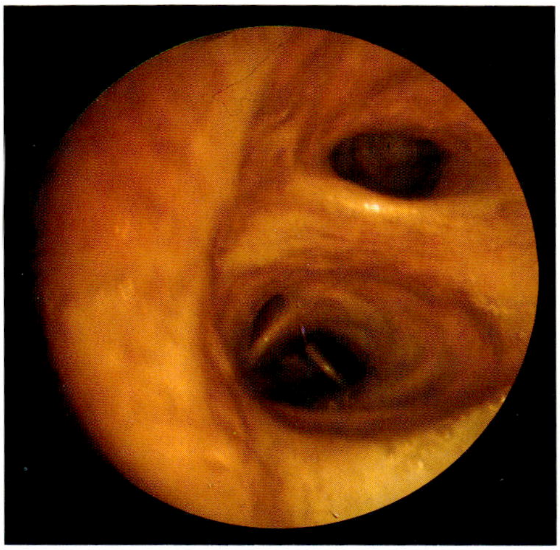

55

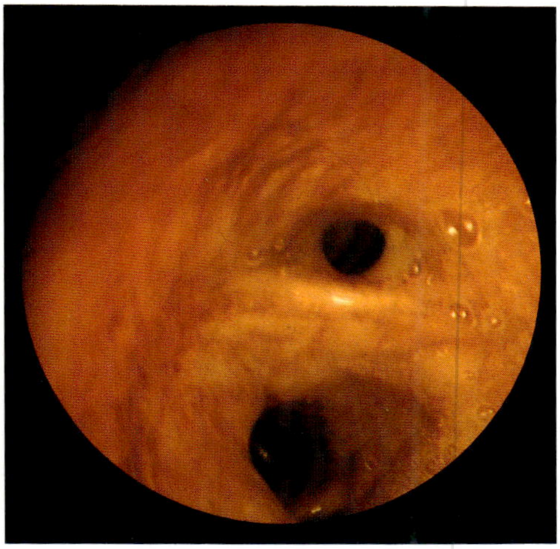

56

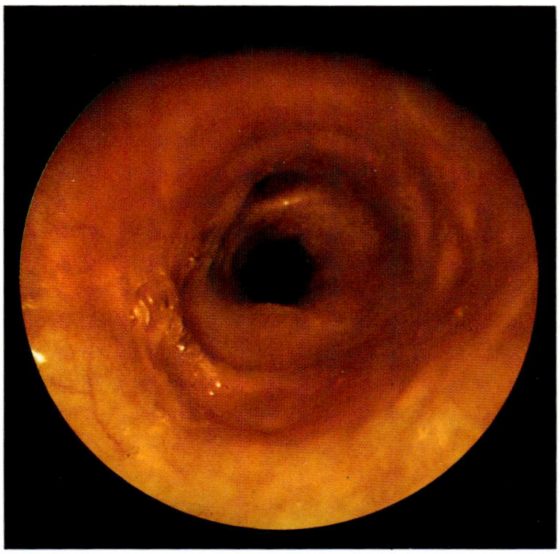

57

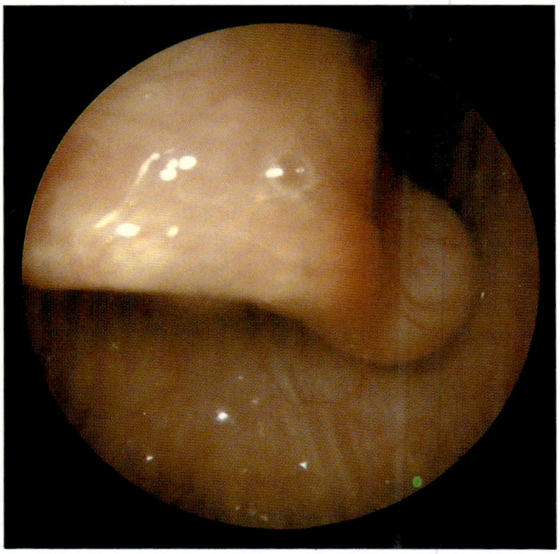

58 Benign "Singers' nodes" on the vocal chords

59a, b (a) A benign papilloma of the larynx situated between the vocal chords. (b) Benign papilloma on right vocal chord

60 Paralysis of the left vocal chord, in which the chord assumes the cadaveric or midline position

61a, b Carcinoma of the larynx protruding from beneath the epiglottis. *1* Epiglottis; *2* tumor

58

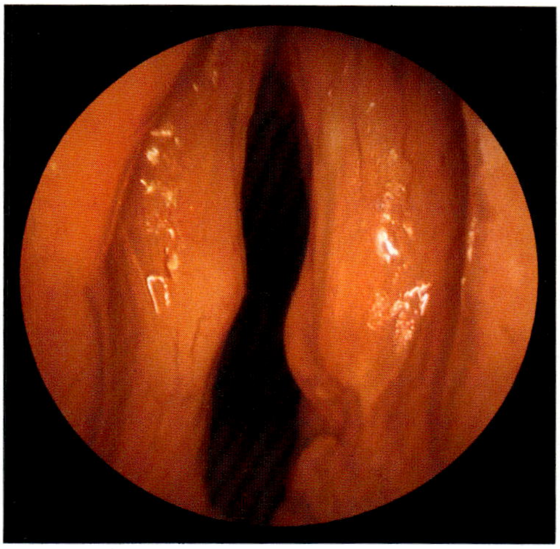

59 a

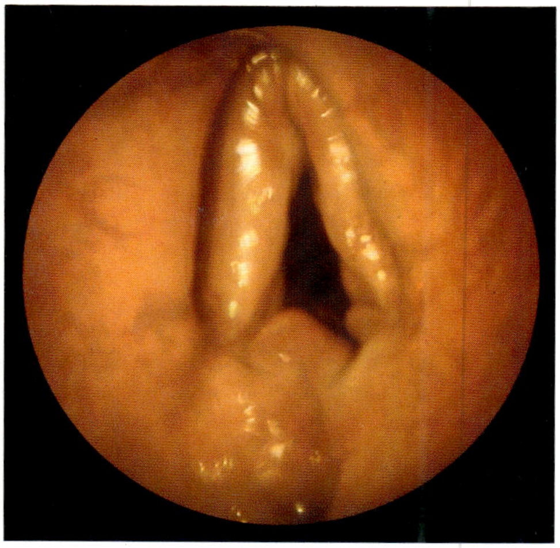

59 b

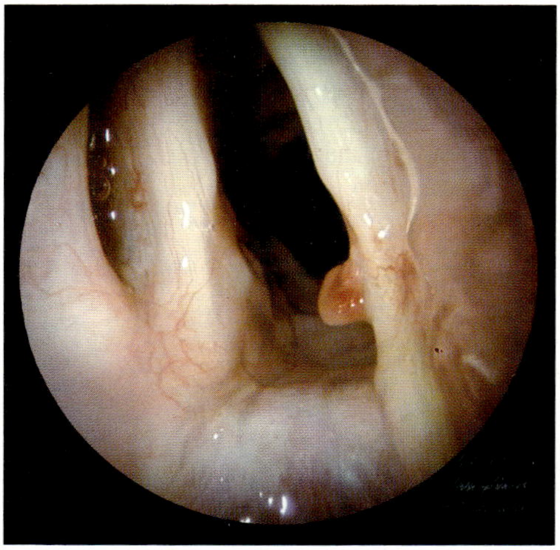

60

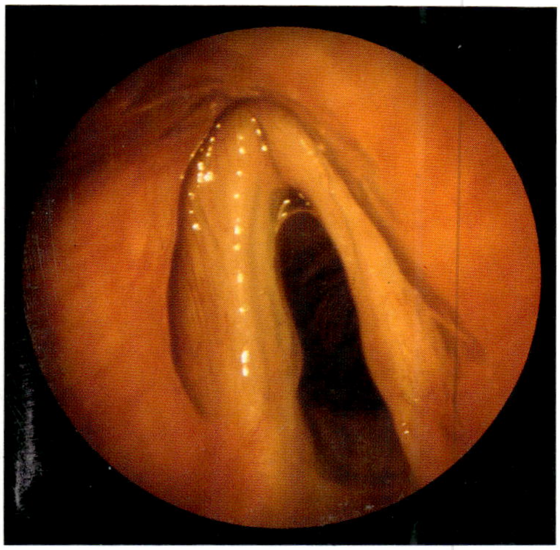

61 a

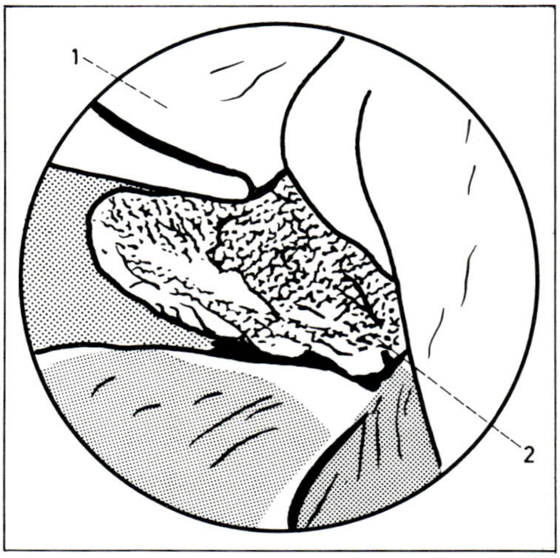


61 b

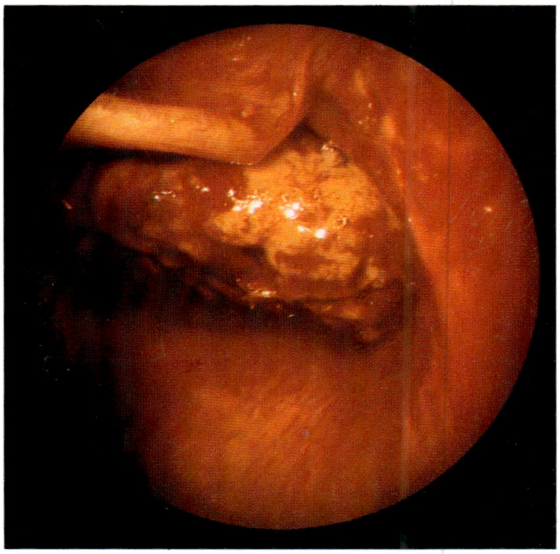

62a, b A view of the cervical trachea with carcinoma of the thyroid infiltrating the wall of the trachea at left. *1* Infiltrating tumor tissue; *2* compressed tracheal cartilage

63 Side-to-side compression of the cervical trachea, exerted by a malignant tumor of the thyroid

64 A primary cancer of the thoracic trachea. Note also the abnormally straight lateral walls of the trachea, giving rise to the triangular deformity which indicates the presence of chronic obstructive-airways disease

65 This is a view of a primary cancer producing narrowing of the intrathoracic trachea. Note the needle tip which has been inserted through the suprasternal notch in order to localize the level of the stenosis

66 A malignant tumor of the right main bronchus just below the level of the carina

62
a

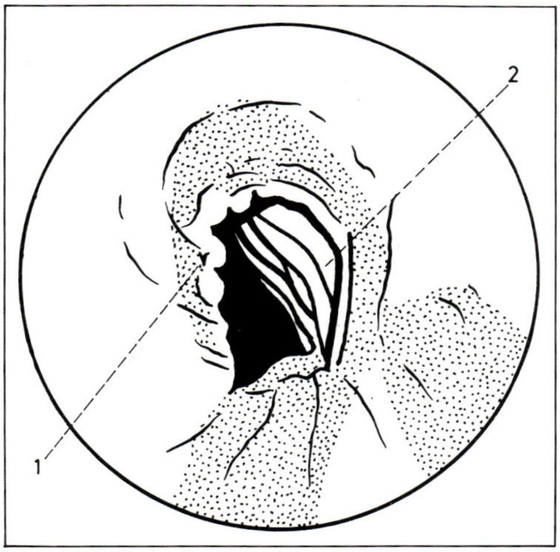


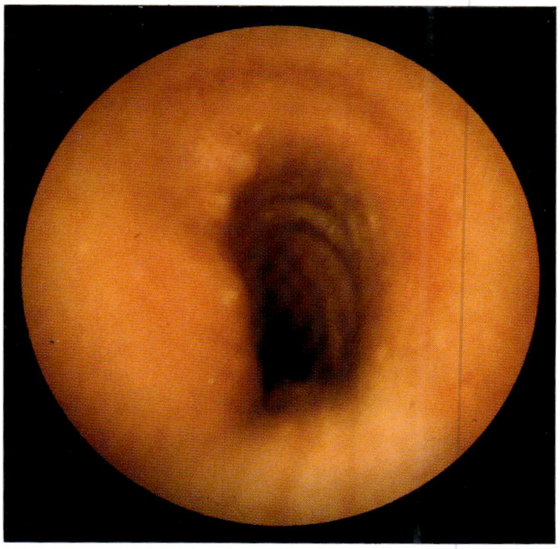

62
b

63

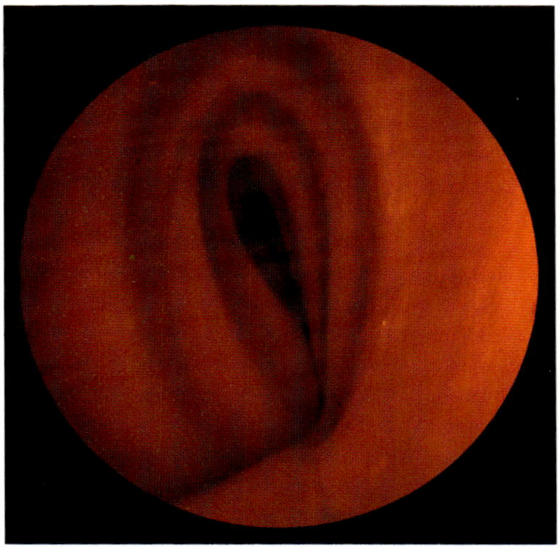

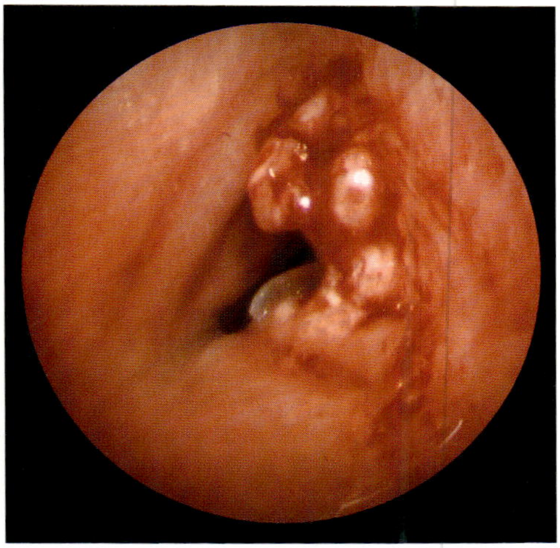

64

65

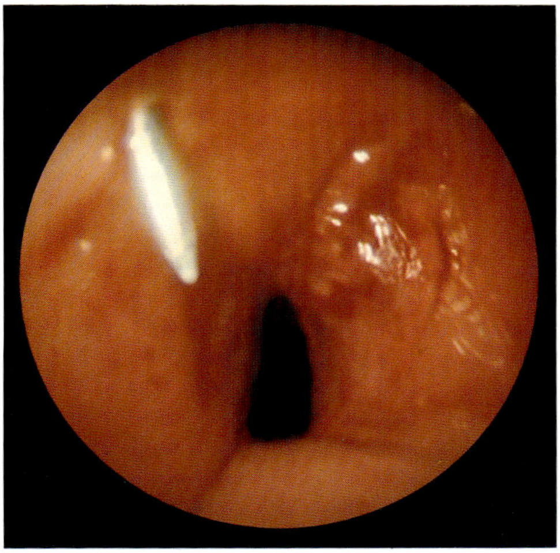

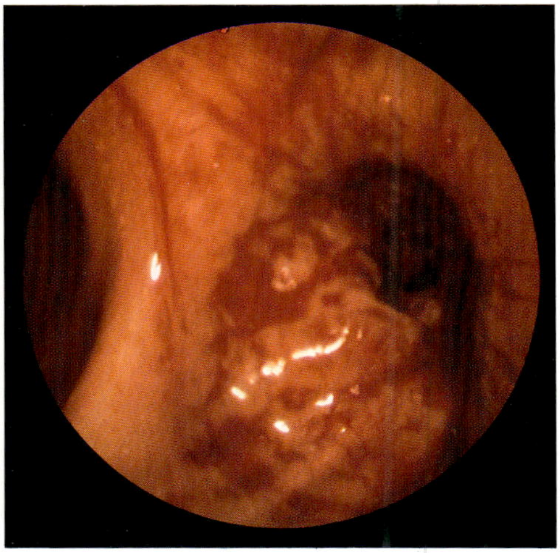

66

67 Carcinoma of the right main bronchus extending up the lateral wall to beyond the carina. Note the extrusion of pus from the affected side, presumably indicating a distal abscess

68 A malignant tumor of the floor of the left main bronchus

69 A tumor of the right main bronchus, producing total occlusion of the lumen

70 Malignant occlusion of the right main bronchus at the level of the carina. Again note the discharge of pus from the opening, indicating a distally situated abscess

71 Malignant growth totally obstructing the lumen of the left upper lobe bronchus. Note the edematous mucosal folds

72 Malignant growth protruding from the right upper lobe bronchus

67

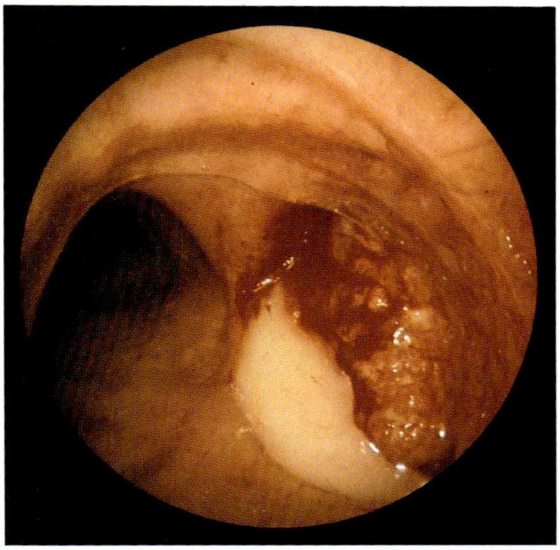

68

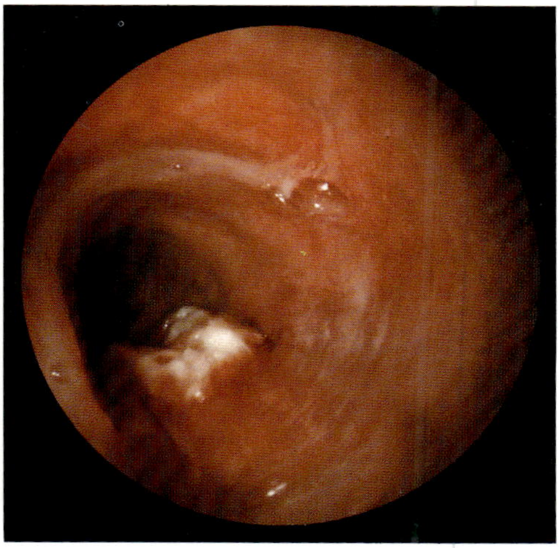

69

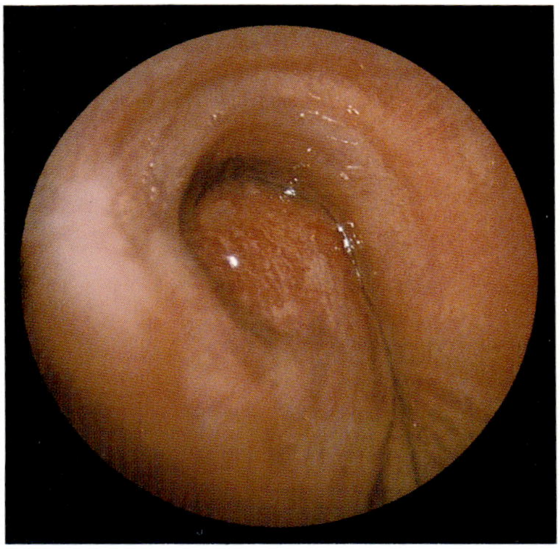

70

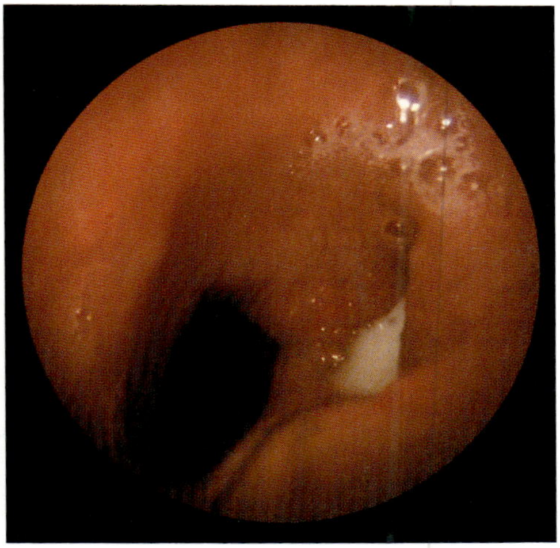

71

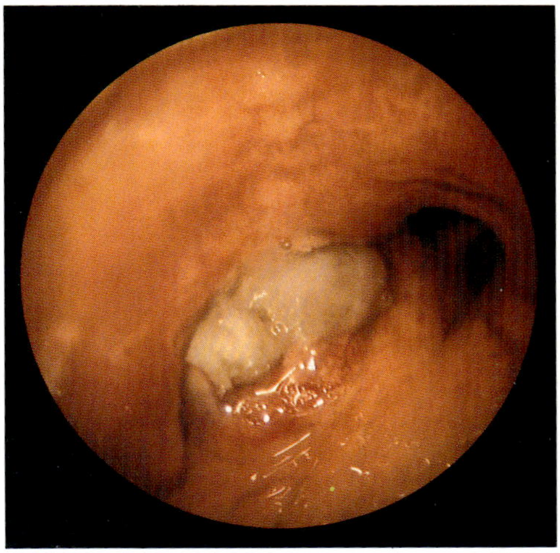

72

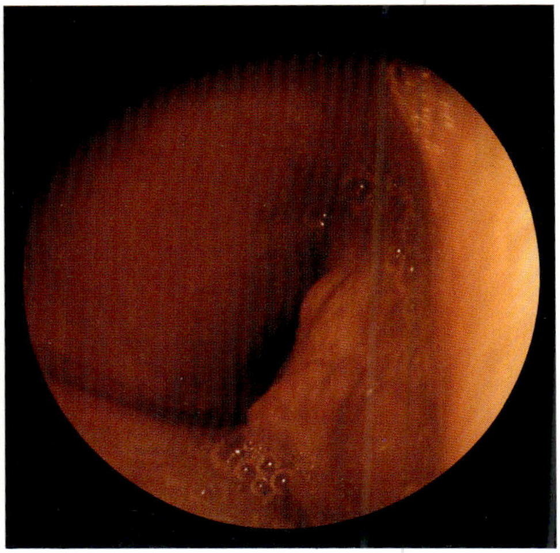

73 A malignant tumor in the opening of the right middle lobe bronchus

74 A tumor outgrowth on the floor of the left upper lobe bronchus. Note the thick edematous spur of the affected bronchus

75a, b Total occlusion of the right upper lobe bronchus by lymph nodes infiltrated by malignant tumor. Note the thickened bronchial spur of the right upper lobe opening and the mucosal corrugations directed into the obstructed orifice. *1* Right intermediate bronchus; *2* thickened, fixed spur of upper lobe opening; *3* occluded opening to right upper lobe; *4* mucosal corrugations

76 Right upper lobe collapse due to endobronchial tumor

77 An adenoma lying in the opening of the right upper lobe bronchus in the patient whose chest radiograph is shown in Fig. 76

73

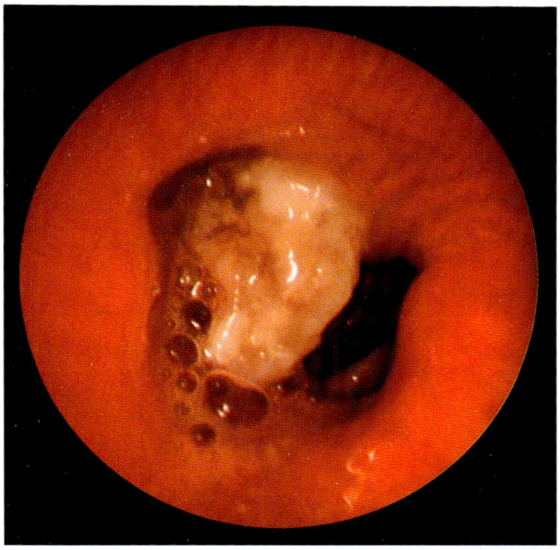

74

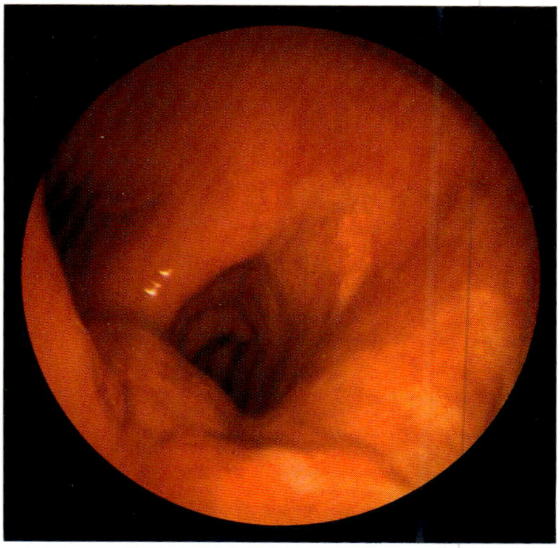

75 a

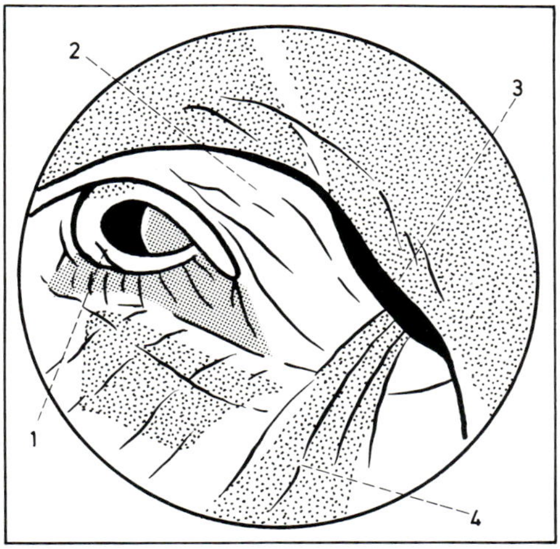


75 b

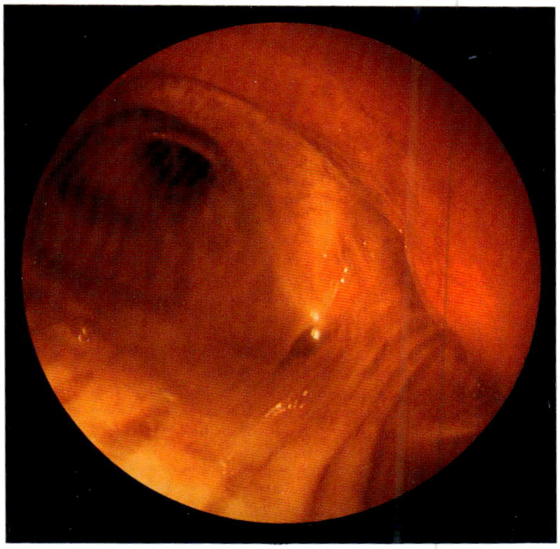

76

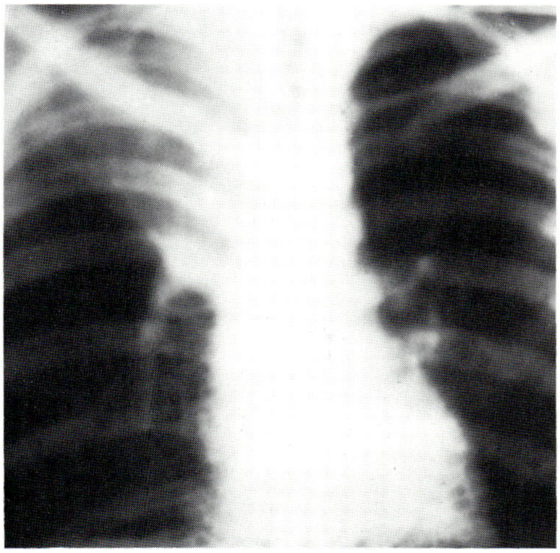

77

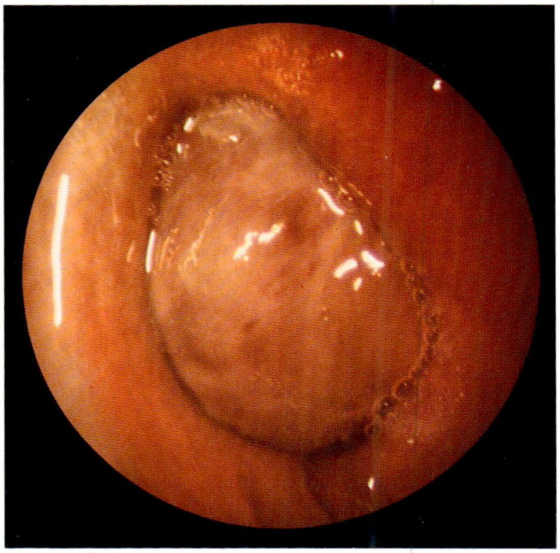

78 Left lower lobe collapse due to endobronchial tumor

79 An adenoma of the left lower lobe bronchus in the patient whose chest radiograph is shown in Fig. 78

80 A thickened malignant carina. Note the broadened anterior extremity and the edema of the surrounding mucous membrane, obscuring the cartilaginous ring structure of the trachea. The carina in this instance did not move with respiration or transmitted cardiac pulsation, nor could it be displaced by means of the bronchoscope tip

81 A broad, malignant carina with associated mucosal edema, resulting in an extension of the thickening toward the posterior extremity of the carina

82 A firm, immobile protrusion of the posterior extremity of the carina produced by malignant infiltrated lymph nodes

83 A primary cancer of the left main bronchus, showing the edematous mucous membrane and thickened, fixed carina

78
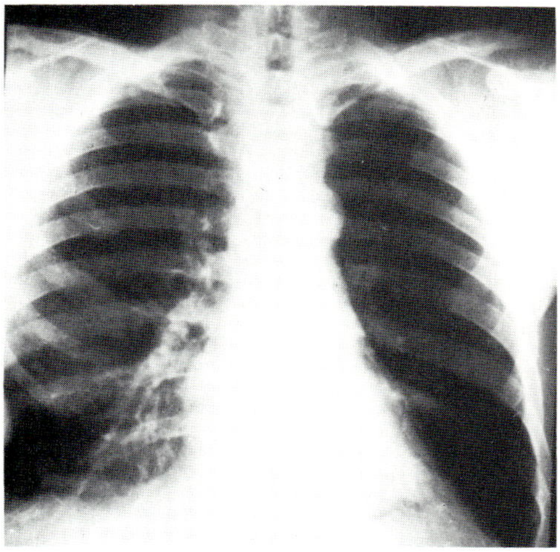

79
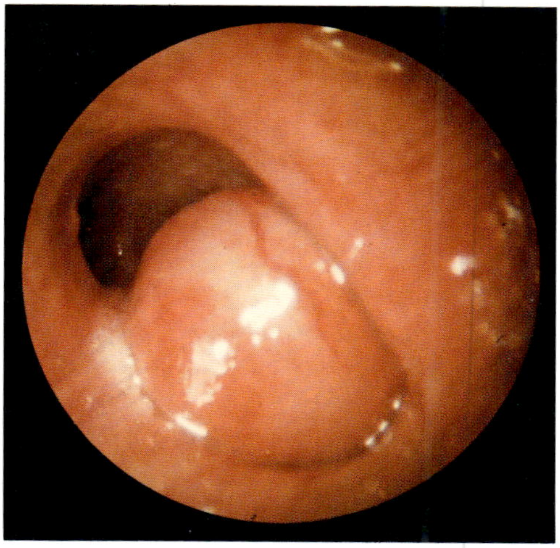

80
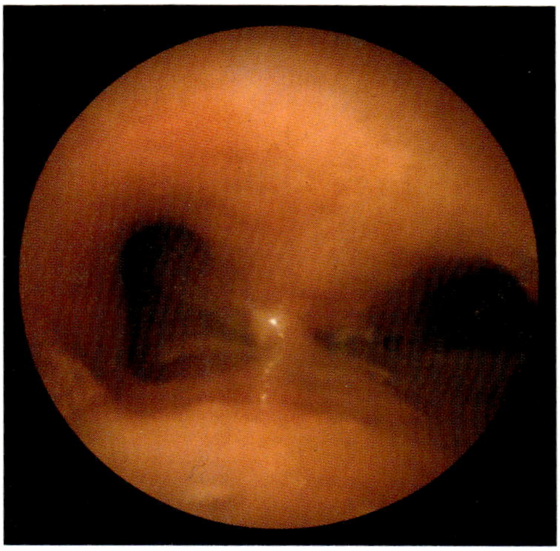

81
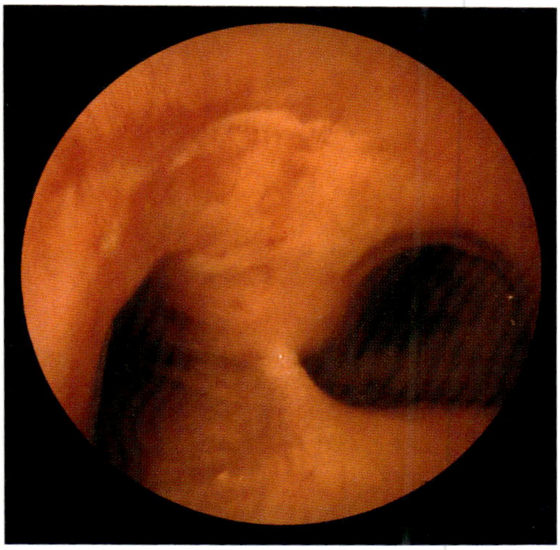

82
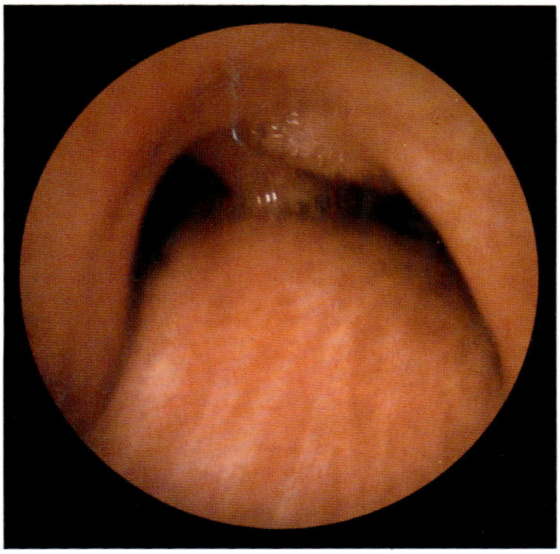

83
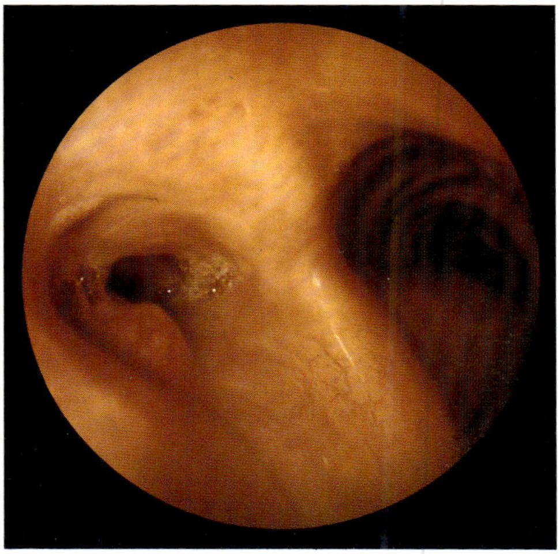

84 A broad, thickened spur of the left upper lobe bronchus. Note the site of a biopsy which provided histological evidence of malignancy

85 A malignant tumor of the right lower lobe with associated thickening of the right upper lobe bronchial spur occasioned by lymph node infiltration

86 A malignant tumor of the right lower lobe with thickening and edema of the mucous membrane caused by peribronchial lymphatic involvement

87 A chest radiograph showing bilateral nodular pulmonary infiltrations

88 Histology of alveolar-cell carcinoma. Specimen collected by means of lung biopsy sampling through the bronchoscope (see text)

89 A catheter manipulated through the opening of the right upper lobe bronchus into the apical segment of this lobe

84

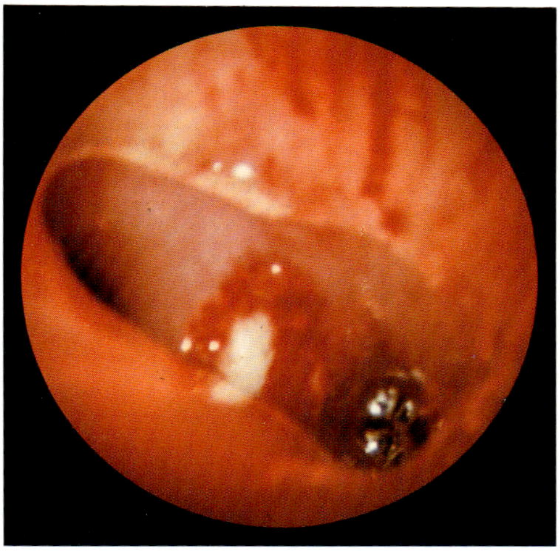

85

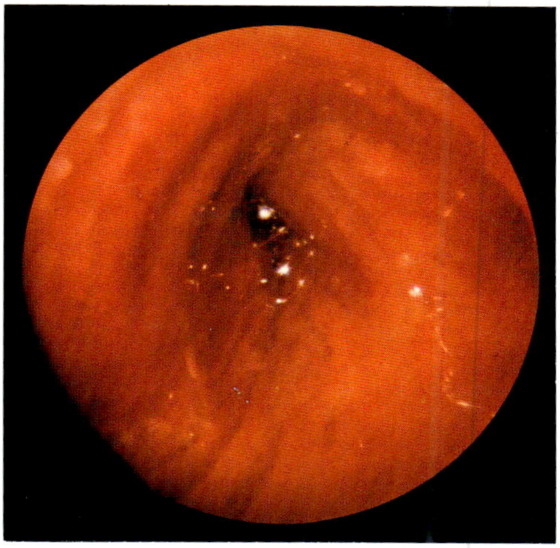

86

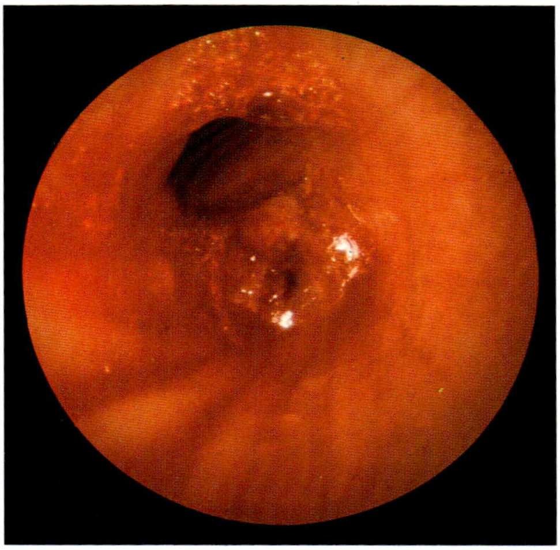

87

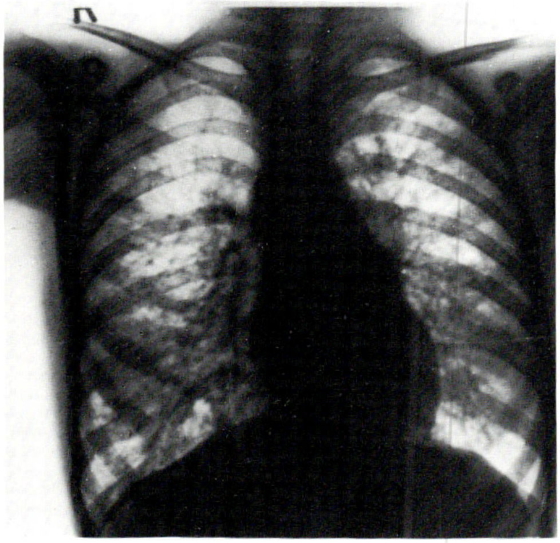

88

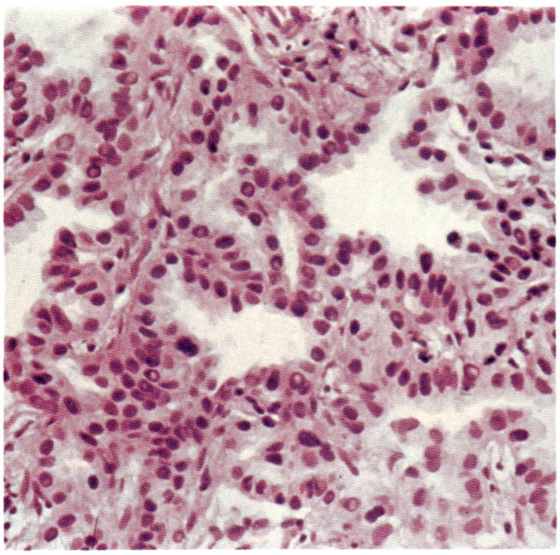

89

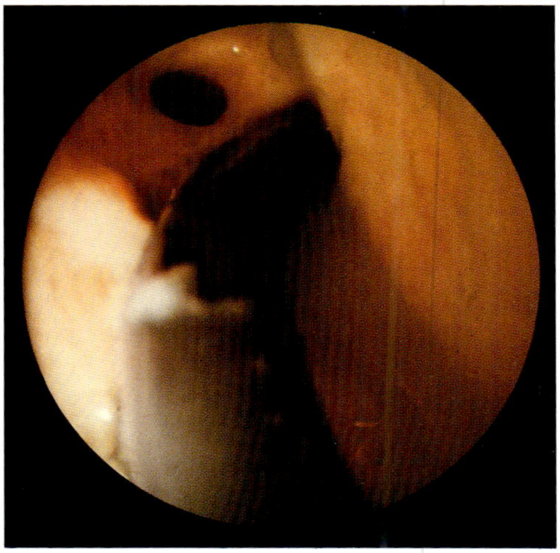

90 a–c (a) A catheter positioned in the right upper lobe apical segment. (b) Catheter positioned in right upper lobe. (c) Catheter in apical segment of right lower lobe

90 a

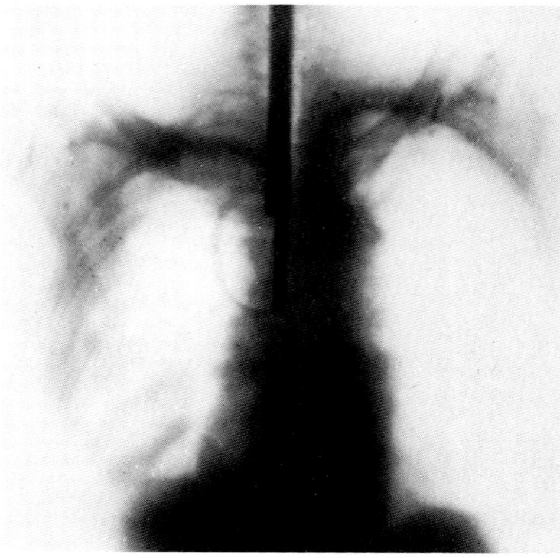

*Trauma of the Airways*

91 a, b Trauma to the larynx caused by an endotracheal tube: stripping of the anterior wall with the avulsed section obstructing the opening between the vocal chords. *1* Opening between vocal chords; *2* area from which the anterior soft tissue wall of the larynx was avulsed; *3* anterior soft-tissue wall of larynx obstructing the opening

92 Severely edematous and hemorrhagic vocal chords of a patient who had, while in a confused state, forcibly removed an endotracheal tube with inflated cuff

93 Pressure necrosis on the posterior ends of the vocal chords due to an endotracheal tube maintained in position

90 b

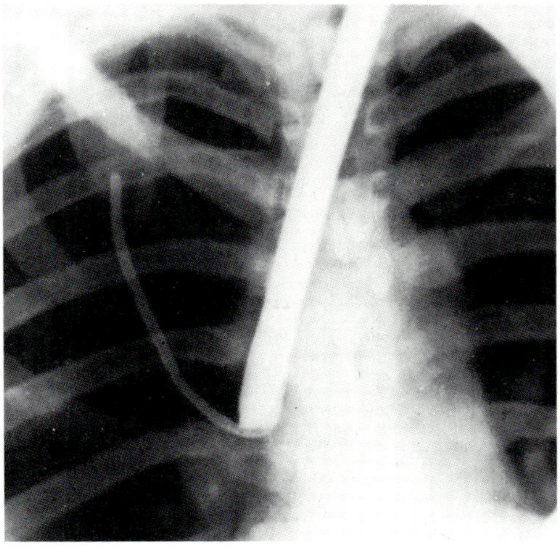

90 c

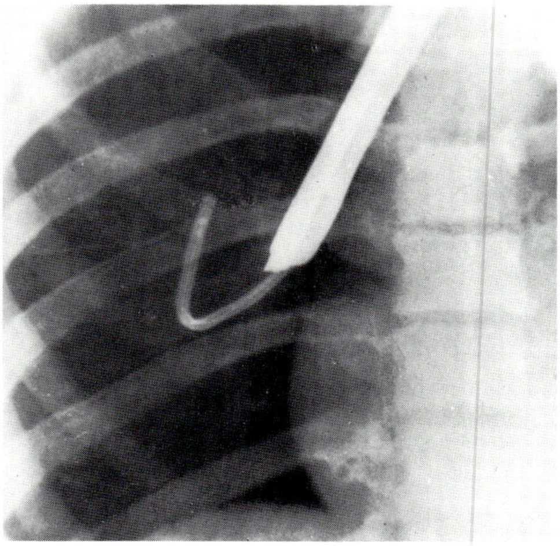

91 a

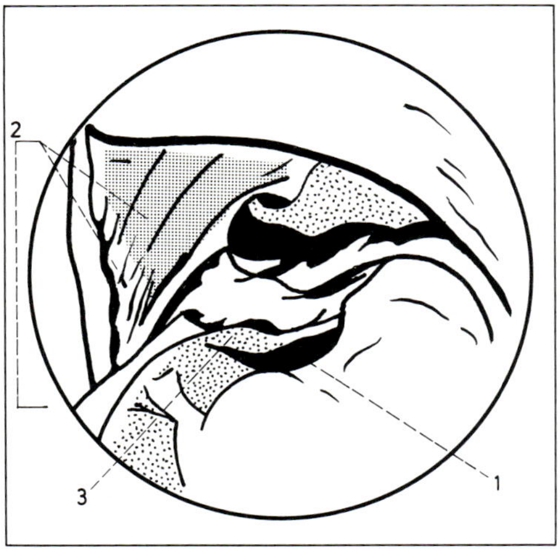


91 b

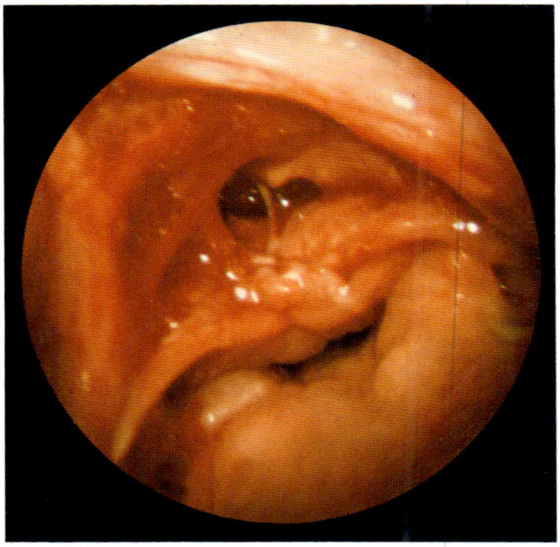

92

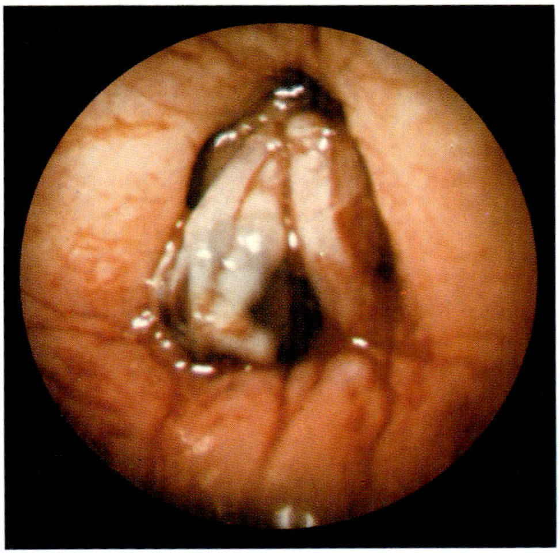

93

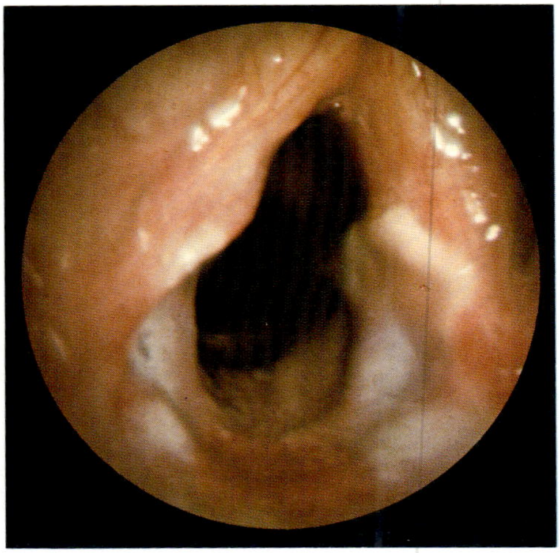

94 A tear in the right main bronchus at the level of the upper lobe bronchus

95 A bronchopleural fistula, the inner opening of which can be seen in the five o'clock position, which developed through sloughing of the suture line of a previously repaired bronchial laceration

96 Severe inflammation and sloughing of the inner wall of the trachea in the area occupied by the inflated cuff of a tracheostomy tube

97 A trachea-esophageal fistula caused by an endotracheal tube. The tracheal opening of the fistula is in the six o'clock position

98 A stenotic lesion with a needle inserted through the tracheal scar to demonstrate that the stenosis corresponds with the level of the original incision

99 A close-up view of a membranous stenosis. Note the normal C-shaped cartilages distal to the stenosis

94

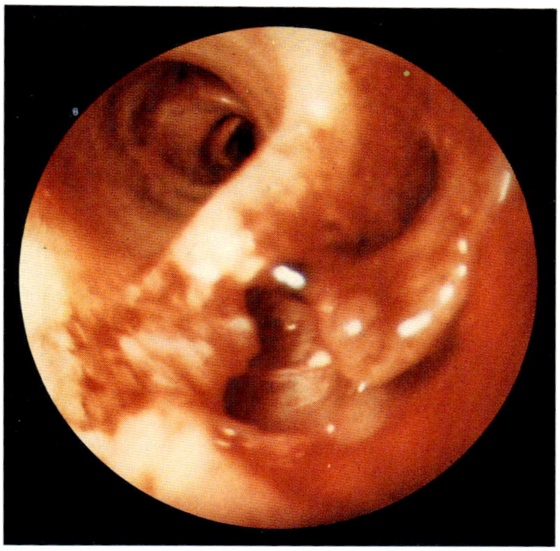

95

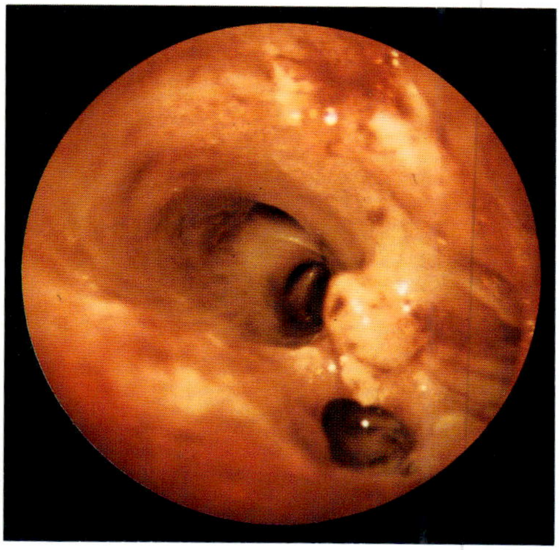

96

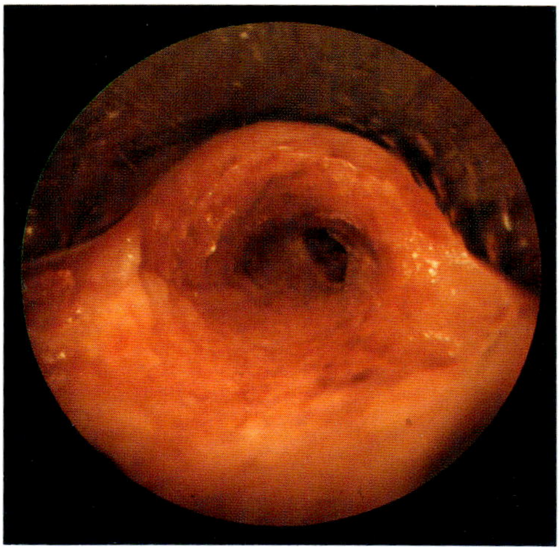

97

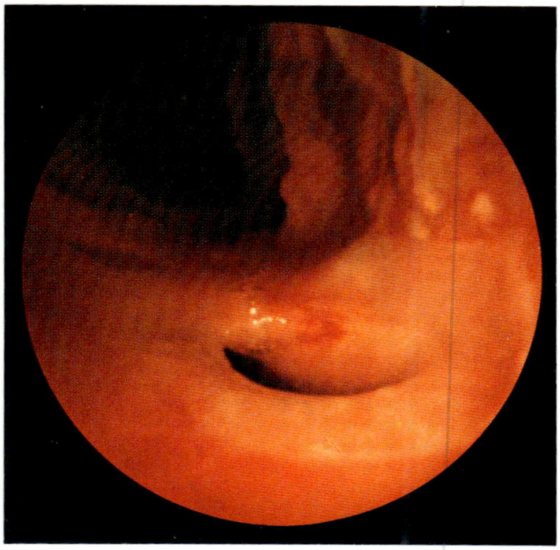

98

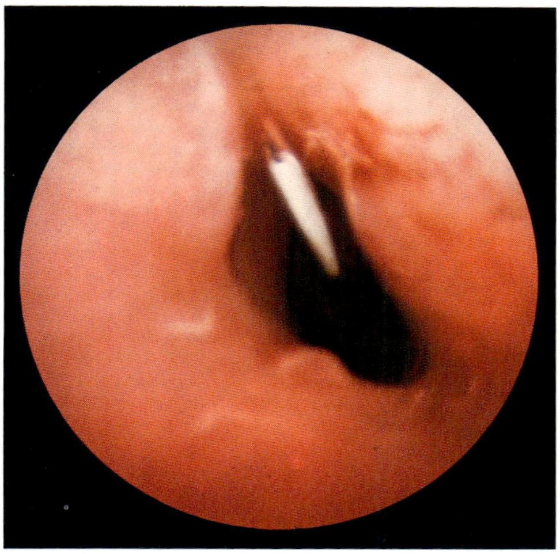

99

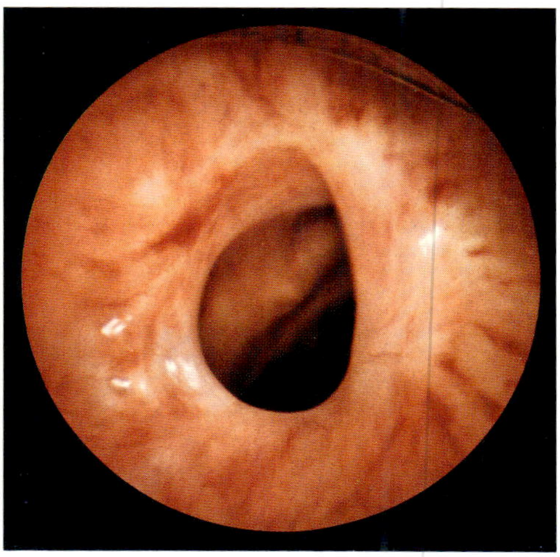

100 A membranous stenosis located distally to the site of the original incision in the tracheal wall marked by the needle

101 Multiple granulomata in the area of the inflated intratracheal cuff. These granulomata may unite to form a stenotic membrane in the trachea

102 Note the granulomata on the left lateral tracheal wall; their organisation may give rise to a membranous stenosis

103 Note the triangular distortion of the cartilage proximal to the membrane projecting from the anterior wall of the trachea

104 A close-up view of the central opening of a membranous stenosis

105 A view of the trachea in the same patient as in Fig. 104, following incision of the stenosing membrane with an electric cautery and dilatation of the tracheal lumen at this point

100

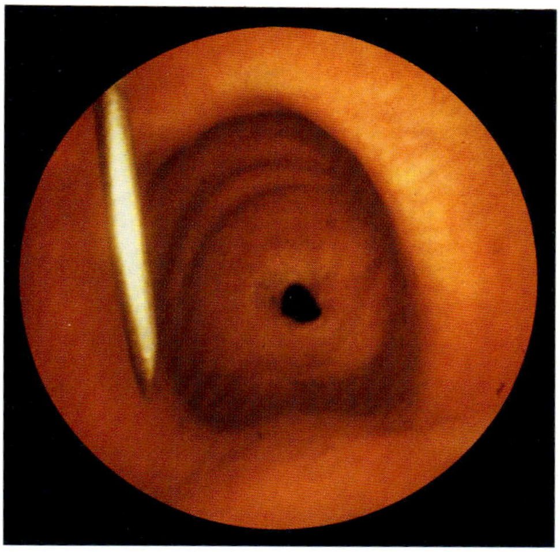

101

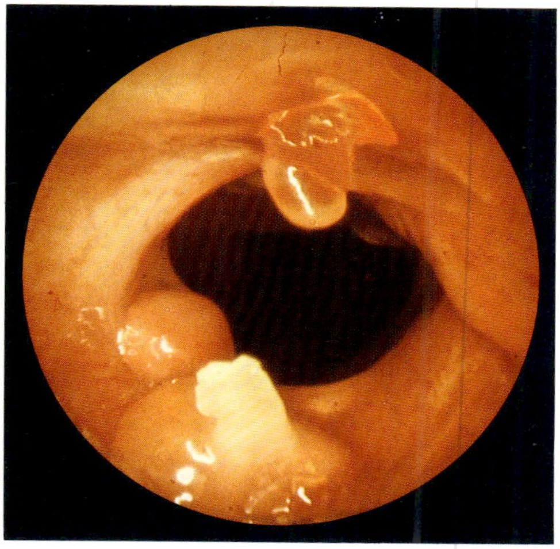

102

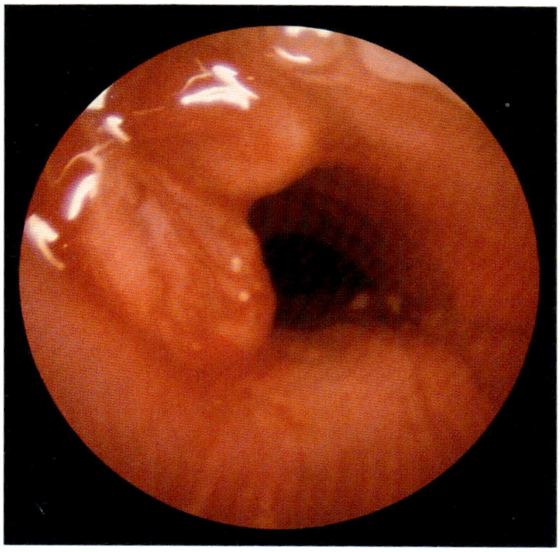

103

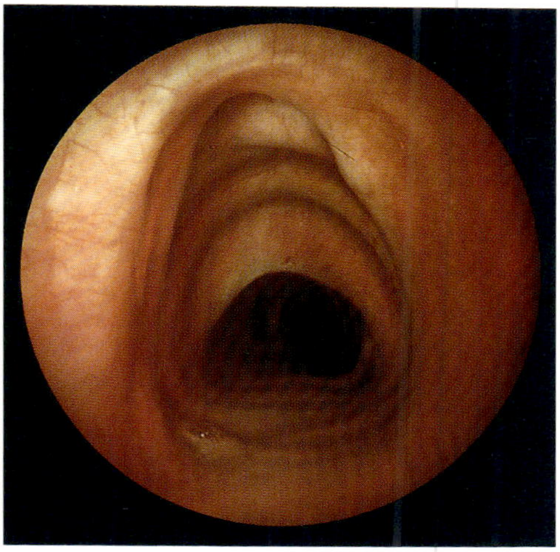

104

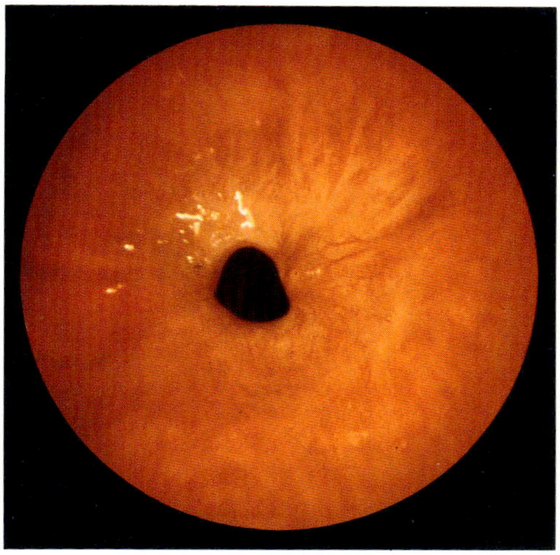

105

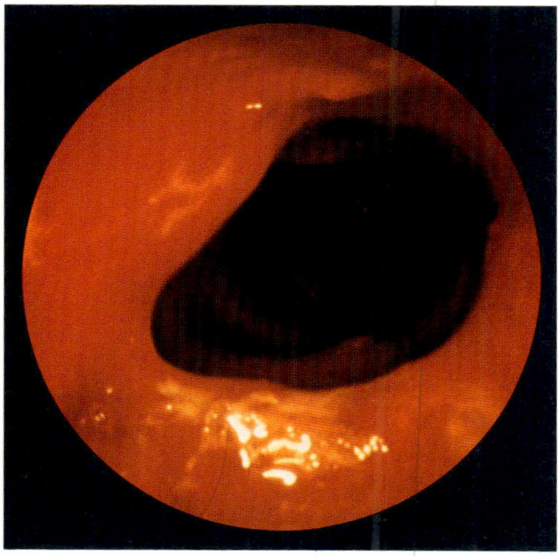

106 The trachea of the same patient as in Fig. 105, showing the end result of dilatation

107 This patient demonstrates that granulomata may re-form after dilatation. Recent tissue growth is seen in the nine o'clock position; it can be removed and the area cauterized directly through the bronchoscope

108 Granulomata in the trachea caused by trauma

*Bronchial Lavage and Postoperative Lobar and Segmental Collapse of the Lungs*

109 A mucous plug obstructing the lower lobe bronchus of the right lung

110 Total left lung collapse caused by obstructing secretions

111 A mucopurulent plug lodged in the left main bronchus of the patient whose chest radiograph is featured in Fig. 110

106

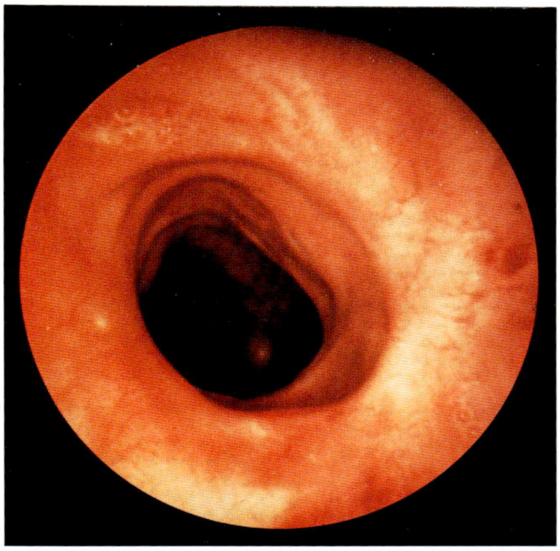

107

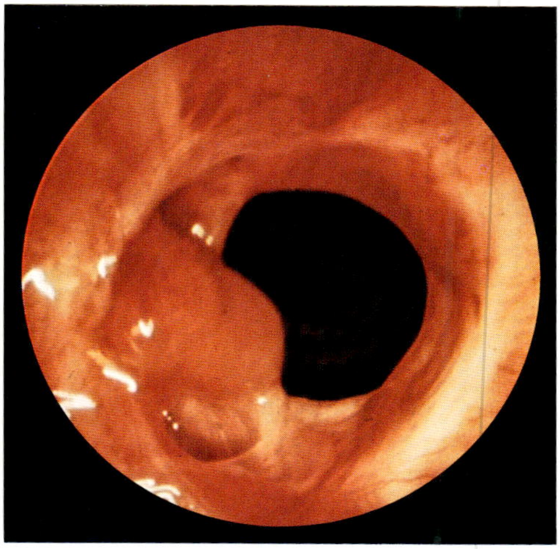

108

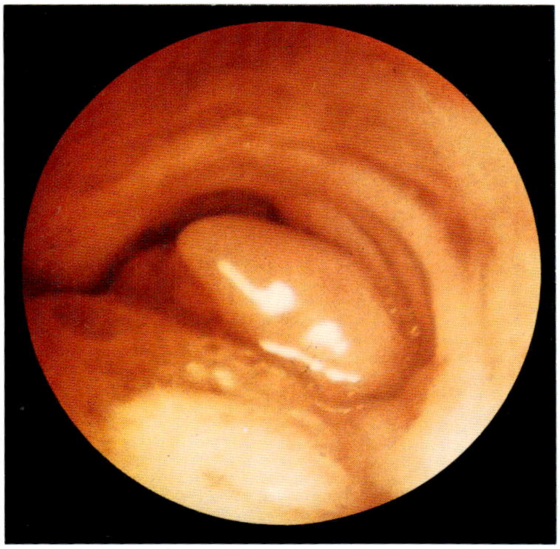

109

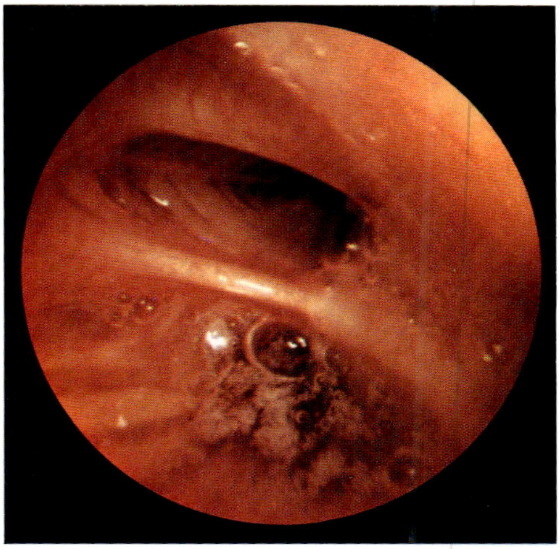

110

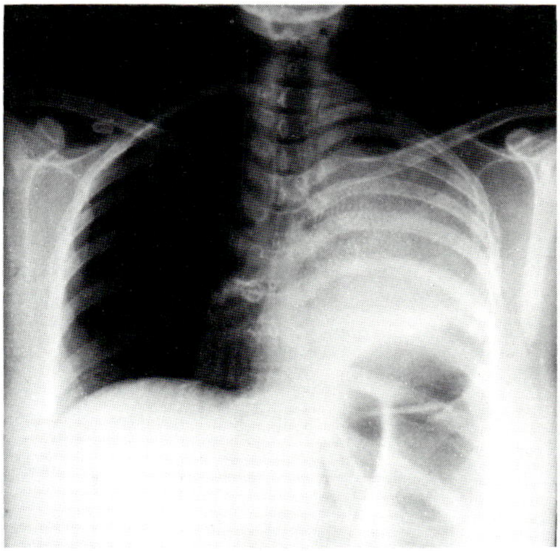

111

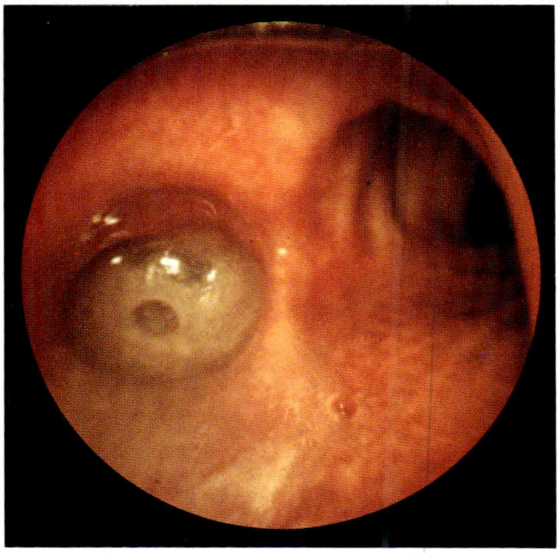

112 The same patient as in Figs. 110 and 111, illustrating the reexpansion of the left lung immediately following removal of the mucopurulent plug and bronchial lavage

113 Right lower lobe collapse due to obstructing secretions

114 In relation to the radiographic appearances in Fig. 113, a mucopurulent plug is shown to obstruct the right lower lobe bronchus of the patient. Note the inflamed and narrowed opening of the right middle lobe bronchus; this narrowing is ascribed to associated bronchospasm

115 Right lower lobe and middle lobe collapse due to obstructing secretions

116 In the patient radiographically illustrated in Fig. 115, a mucopurulent plug is seen to obstruct the intermediate bronchus on the right. Note the thickened, inflamed spur of the right upper lobe bronchus

117 This radiograph demonstrates the reexpansion of the right lower and middle lobes following removal of the mucopurulent plug in the patient described in Figs. 115 and 116

112

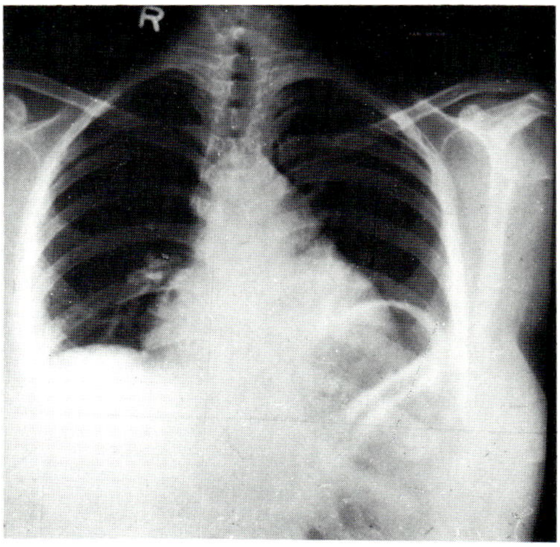


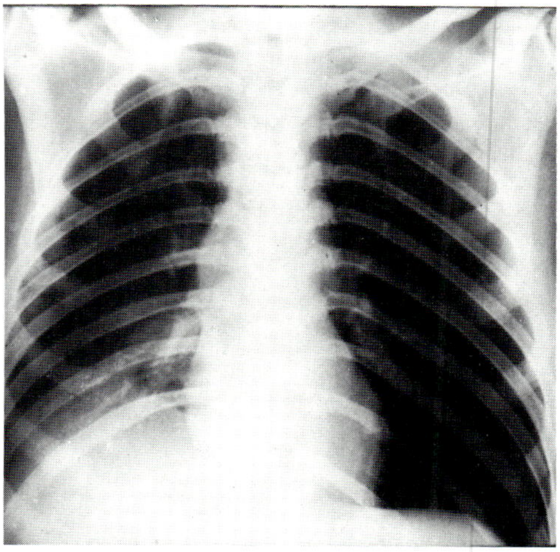

113

114

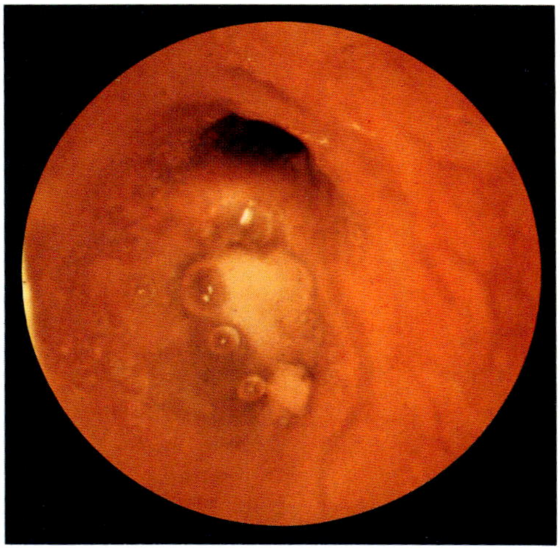

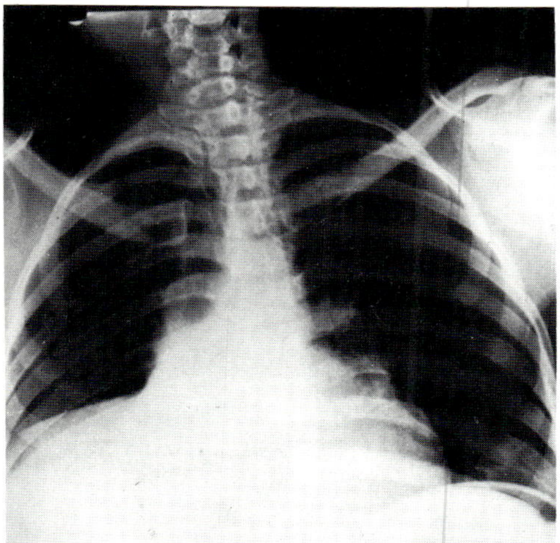

115

116

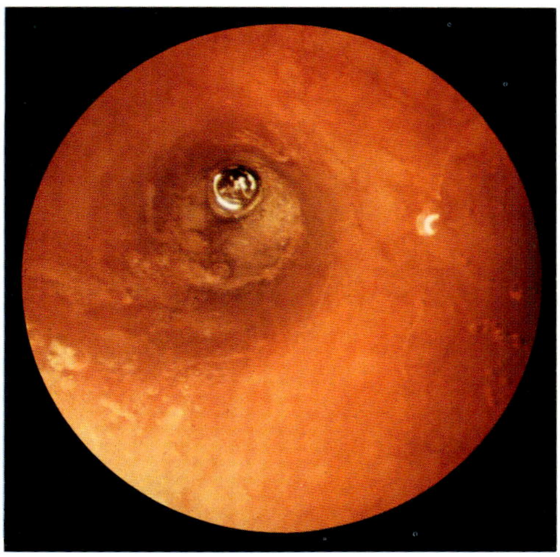

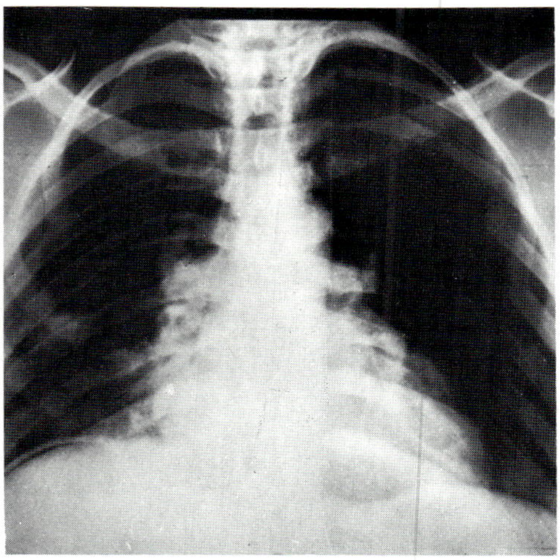

117

118 Total left lung collapse. On bronchoscopic examination no definite secretory plug could be identified, although large quantities of mucopurulent secretions were present

119 Reexpansion of the left lung following bronchial lavage in the patient featured in Fig. 118

120 Total right lung collapse in an infant. On bronchoscopy no definite plug could be seen, but mucopurulent secretions were removed by bronchial lavage

121 Following bronchial lavage in the infant described in Fig. 120, satisfactory reexpansion of the right lung is observed

122 Right upper lobe collapse in a patient with tracheostomy and intermittent positive pressure ventilation

123 Catheterization of the right upper lobe via a bronchoscope passed through the tracheostomy wound

18

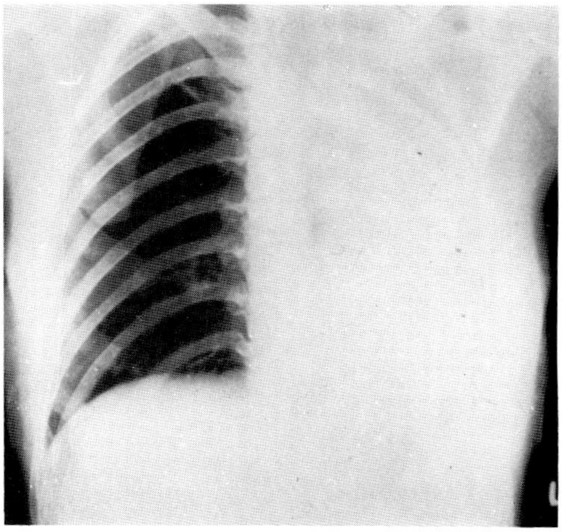

119

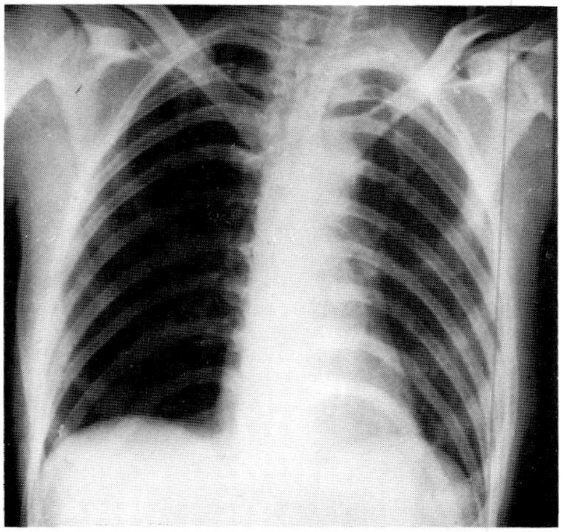

20

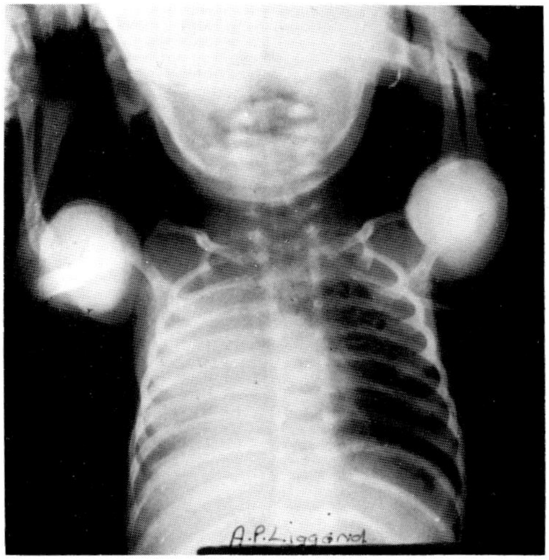

121

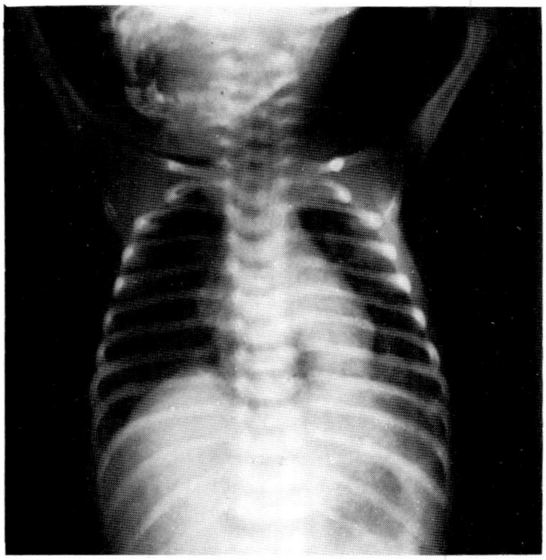

22

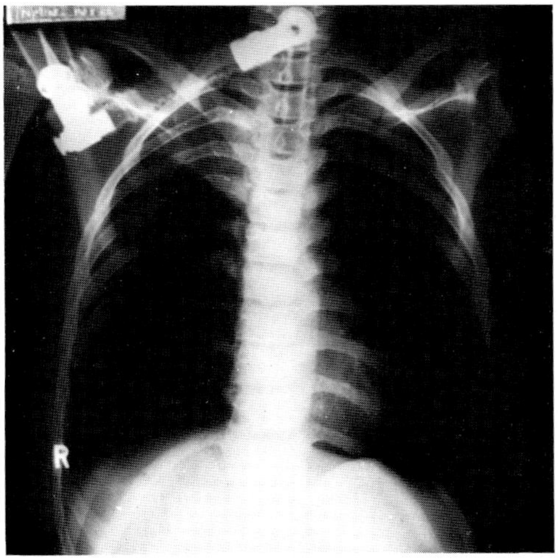

123

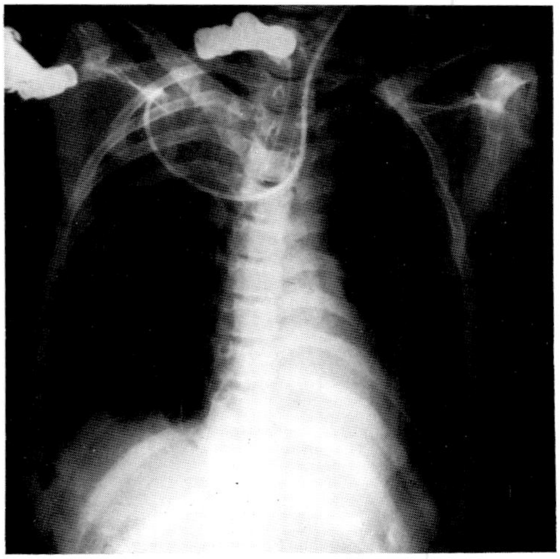

24

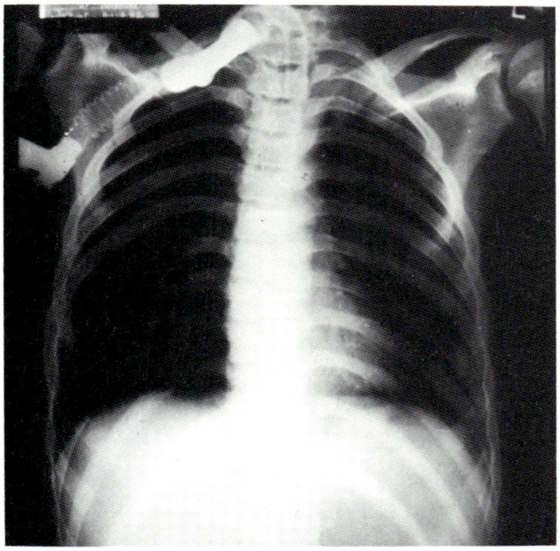

125

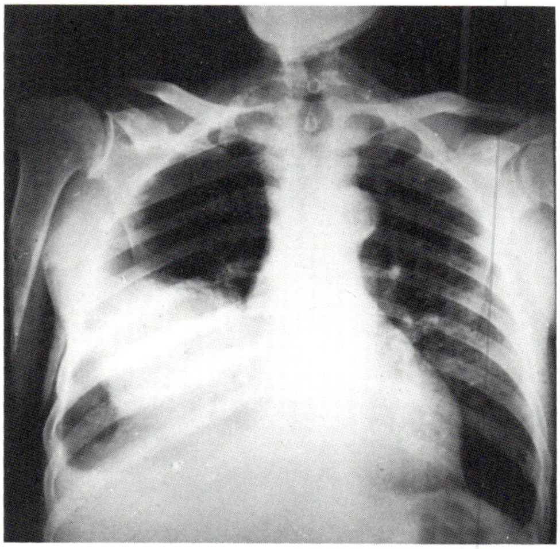

126

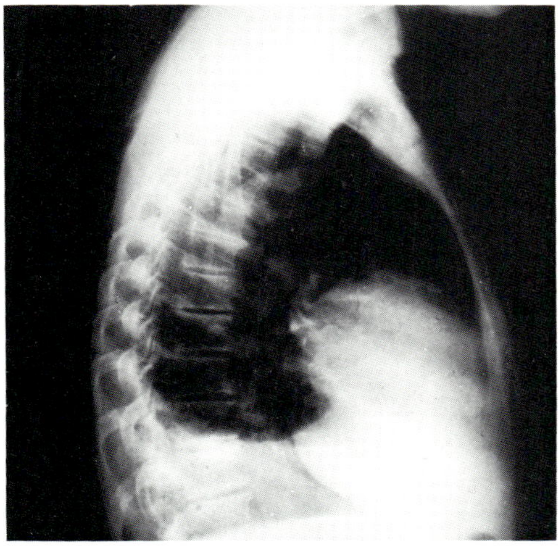

127

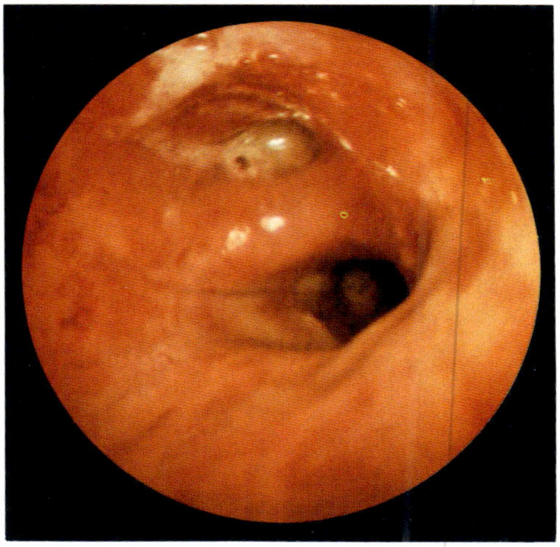

128

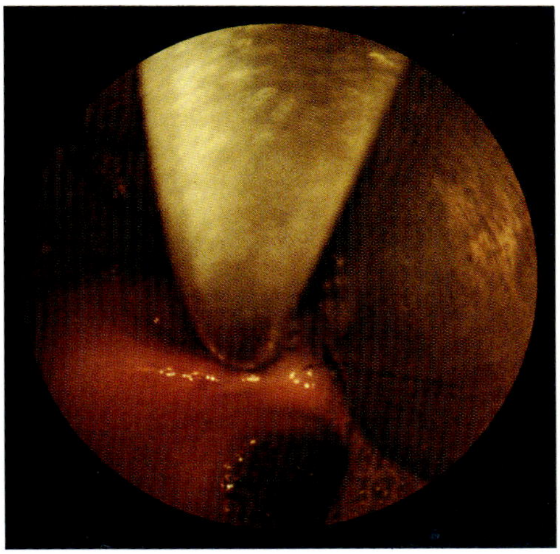

129

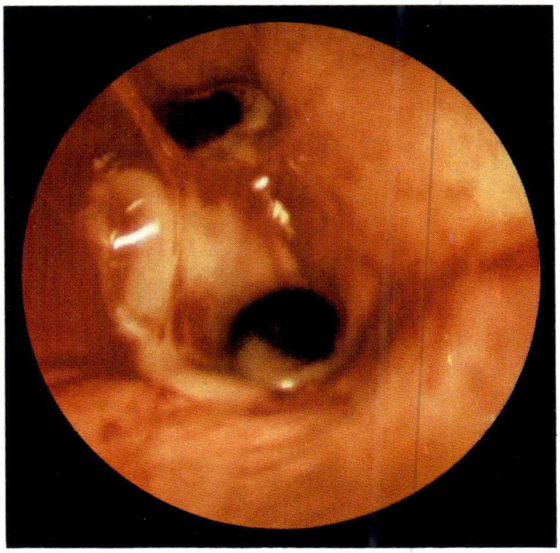

130 Radiological improvement of the abscess following catheterization in the patient illustrated in Figs. 125 and 126

131, 132 Selective catheterization of the right middle lobe bronchus, showing bronchiectasis and parenchymal destruction of the lobe

*Tuberculosis Involving the Airways*

133 The right main bronchus viewed at the level of the middle lobe bronchus, showing a side-to-side narrowing of the lower lobe bronchus caused by tuberculous lymph nodes, plus occlusion of the middle lobe bronchus

134, 135 Right middle lobe collapse due to enlarged tuberculous lymph nodes

30

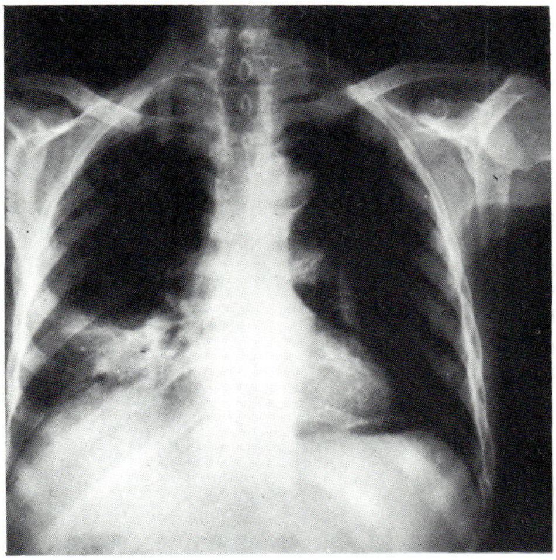

131

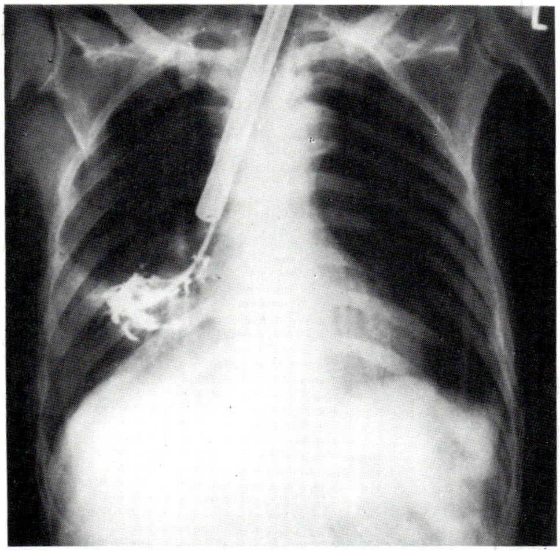

32

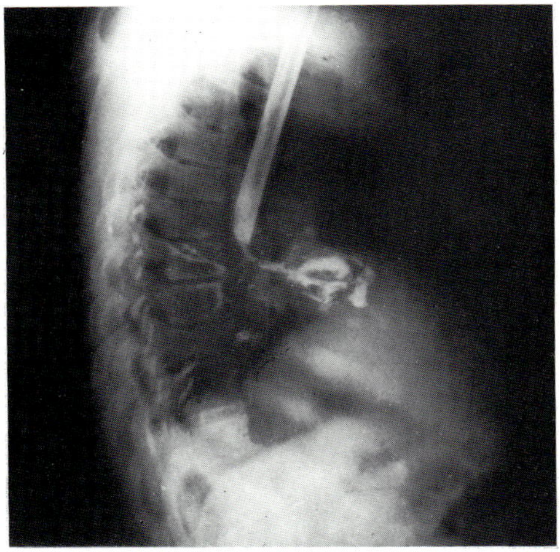

133

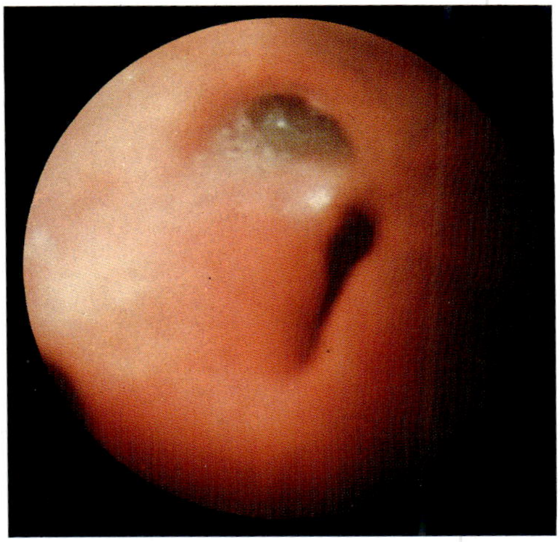

134

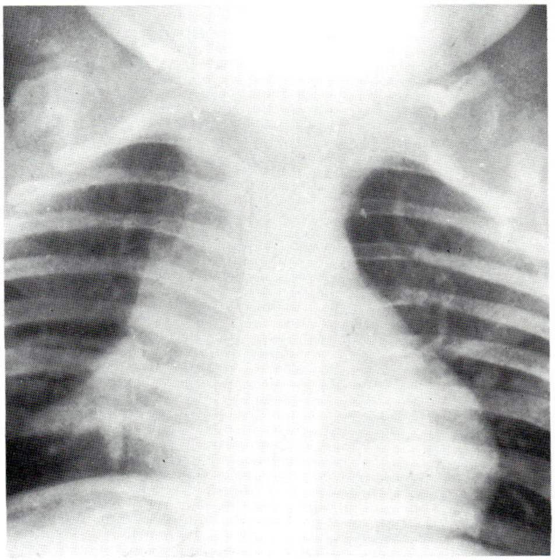

135

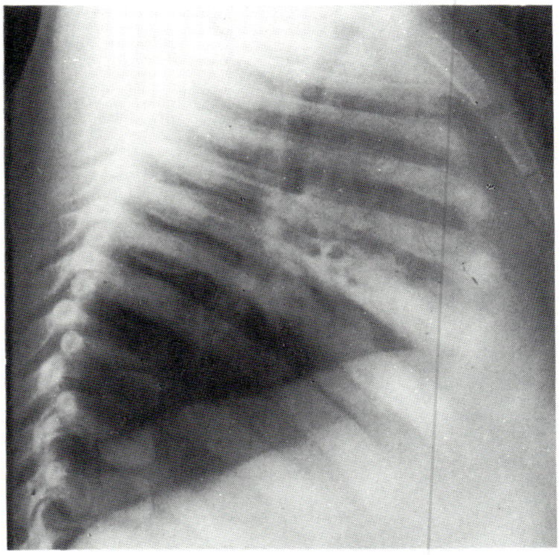

136 In the same patient featured in Figs. 134 and 135, the eruption of a tuberculous lymph node into the bronchial lumen is demonstrated. On account of the distortion of bronchial contours produced by the enlarged surrounding nodes, the right middle lobe bronchial opening could not be visualized, nor could this bronchus be filled with contrast media

137 An enlarged right hilar lymph node

138 In the same patient as in Fig. 137, the thickened, fixed spur of the right upper lobe bronchus and the partial obstruction of the bronchial orifice are demonstrated. A lymph node removed at mediastinoscopy showed evidence of tuberculosis

139 Total collapse of the right lower lobe in a patient with healed intrabronchial tuberculosis

140 Pinpoint stenosis of the intermediate bronchus immediately below the opening to the upper lobe bronchus in the patient featured in Fig. 139

141 Isolated stenosis of the right middle lobe bronchus, probably the result of healed tuberculosis

36

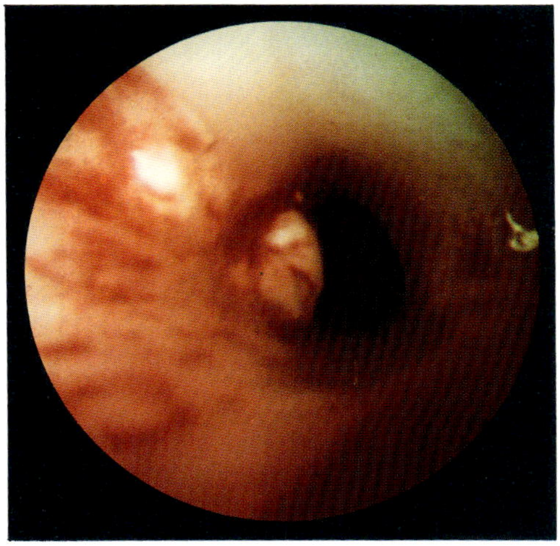

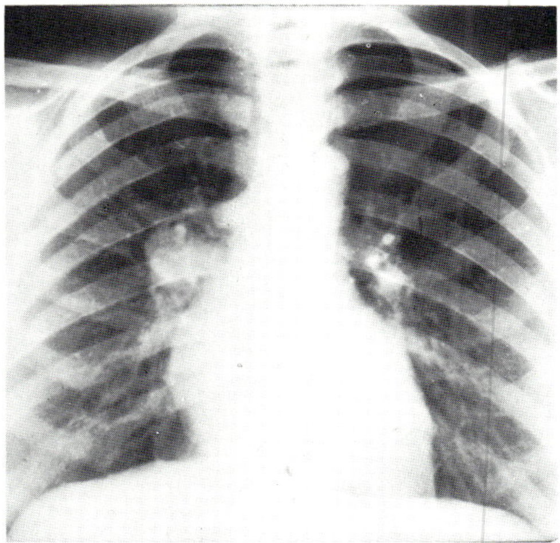

137

38

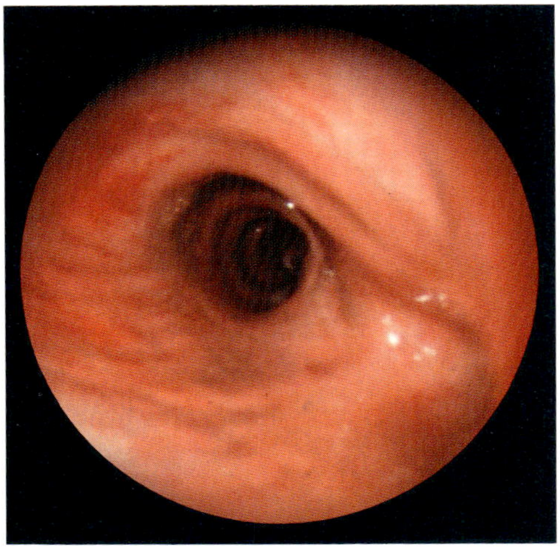

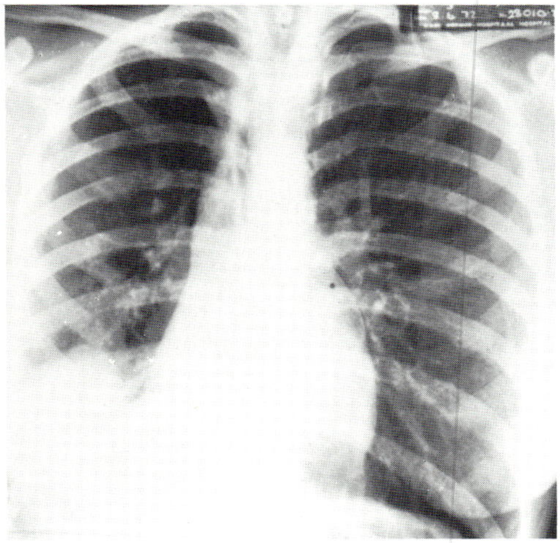

139

40

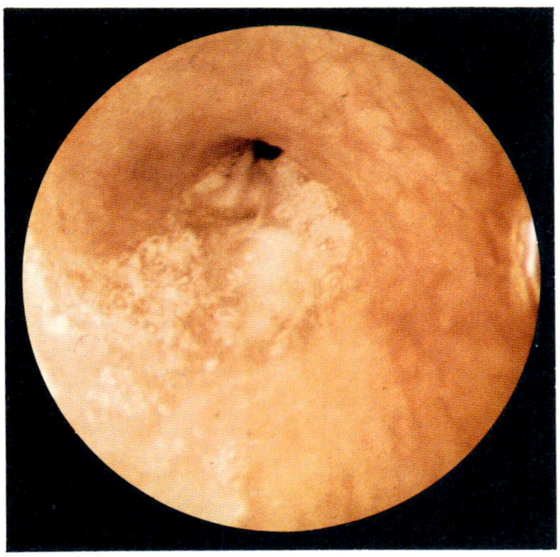

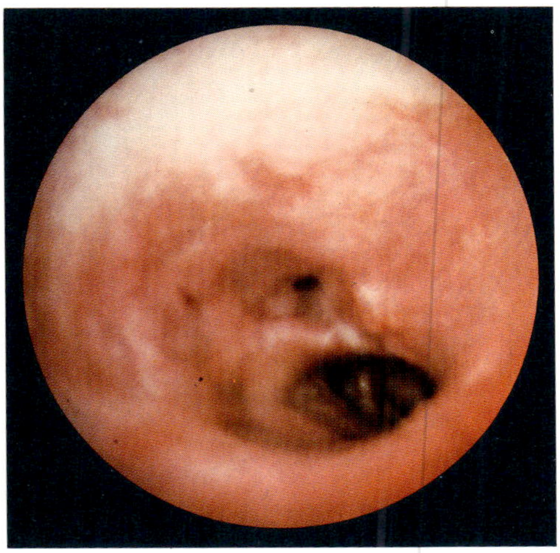

141

142 Occlusion of the right middle lobe bronchus with associated distortion of the right main bronchus, probably the result of healed tuberculosis

143 A thickened, edematous epiglottis in association with tuberculous laryngitis

144 Caseating tuberculous laryngitis

145 Caseating tuberculosis involving the intrathoracic trachea and the carina

146 The lower end of the trachea and the carina of a patient with primary amyloid of the airways. Note the thickening of the mucous membrane and the nodules on the carina

147 The left main bronchus of the same patient as in Fig. 146, displaying a cherry-red tumor of the bronchial wall at the level of the left upper lobe bronchial opening. This tumor mass was found to consist of an amyloid infiltration of the mucosal tissue

142

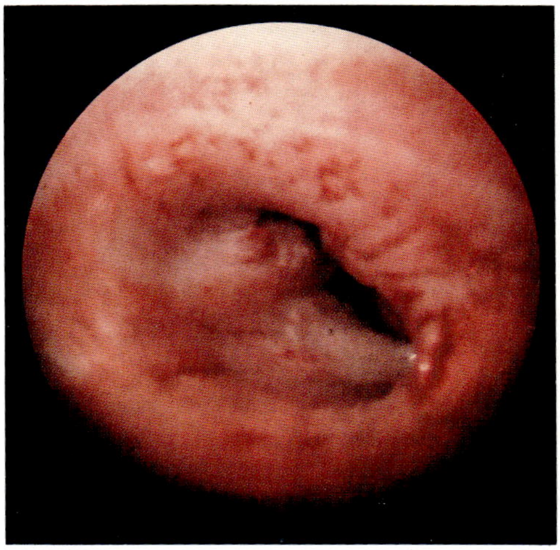

143

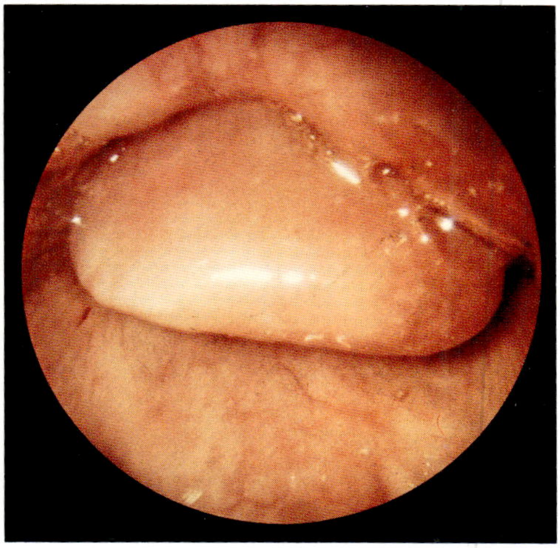

144

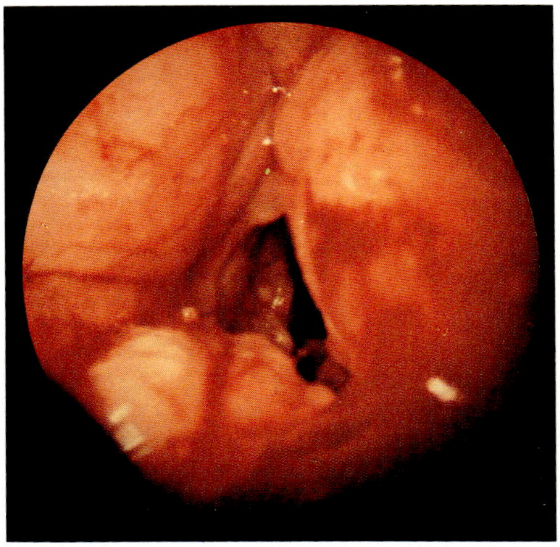

145

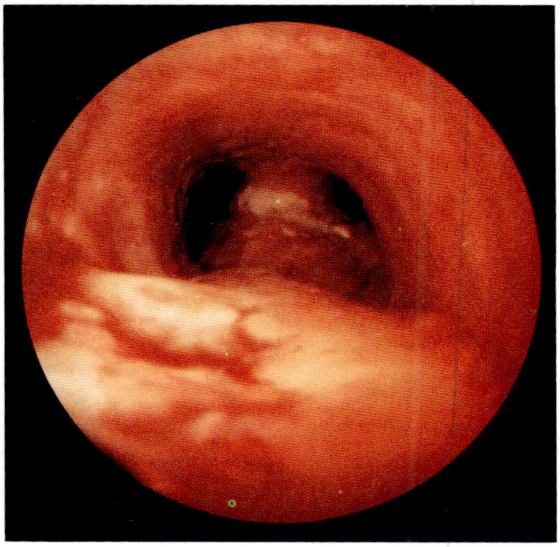

146

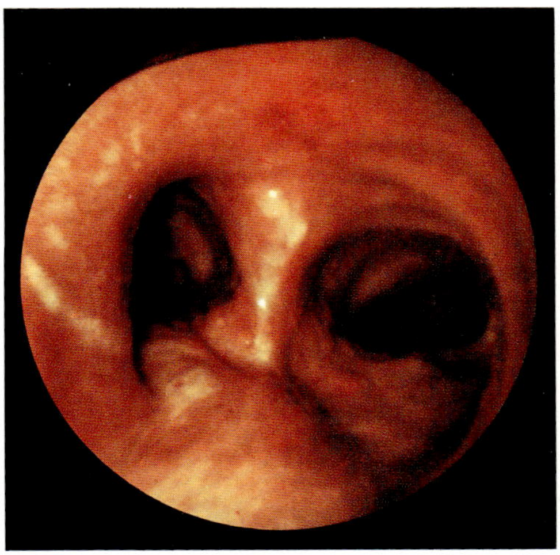

147

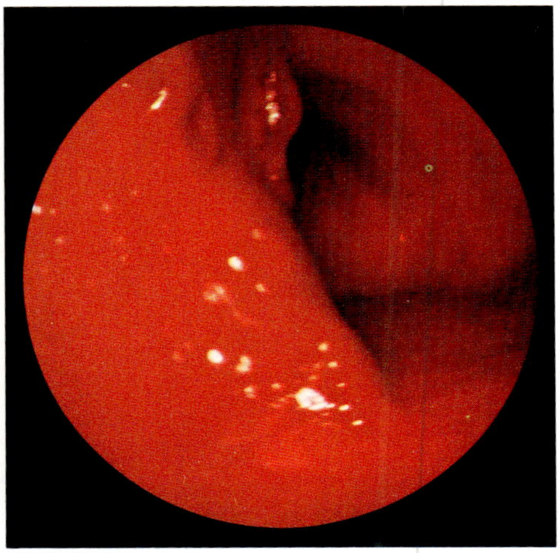

148 Right main bronchus showing prominent mucosal corrugations on the posterior membrane

149 Granulomatous mucous membrane showing fragmented particles of purulent mucus, a common finding in the chronic bronchitic subject or heavy smoker

150 The appearances of acute bronchitis include mucopurulent secretions and inflammatory erythema of the mucous membrane, which may be ascribed in part to persistent coughing

151 A turgid, blunted spur of the left upper lobe bronchial orifice in relation to an acute inflammatory process

152 Acute bronchitis with swollen mucous membrane and mucopurulent secretions. Note the narrowed lumen of the right main bronchus; this narrowing has been produced by a combination of inflammatory swelling of the mucous membrane and associated bronchospasm

153 Chronic bronchitis with hemorrhagic mucous membrane and narrowing of the basal segmental bronchi due to bronchospasm

148

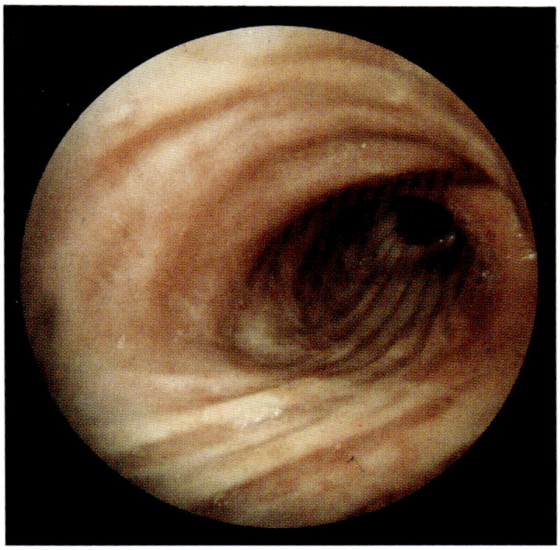

149

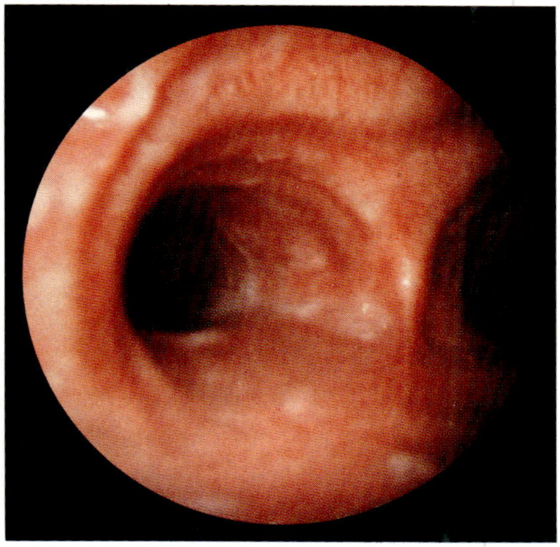

150

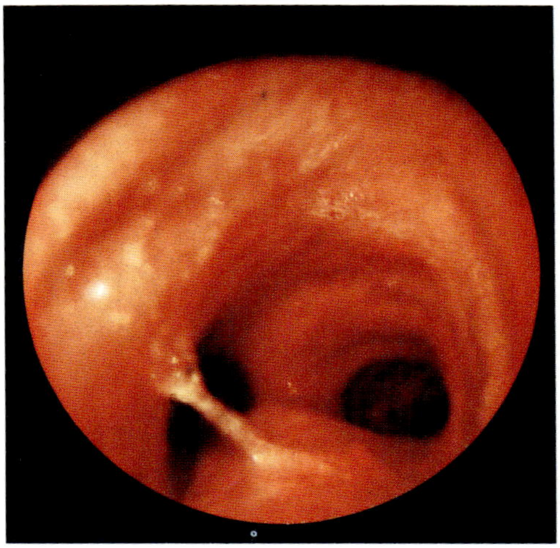

151

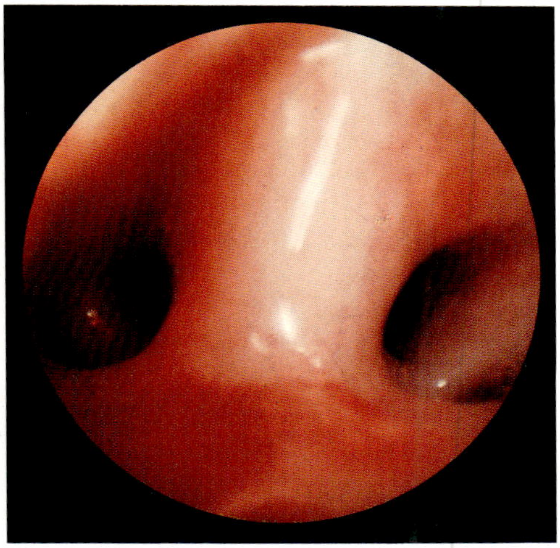

152

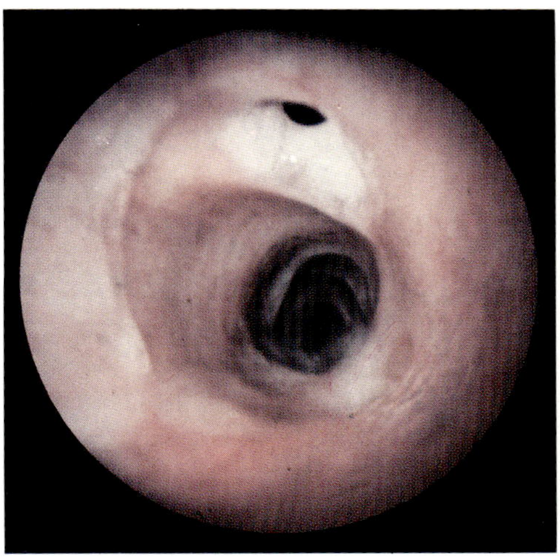

153

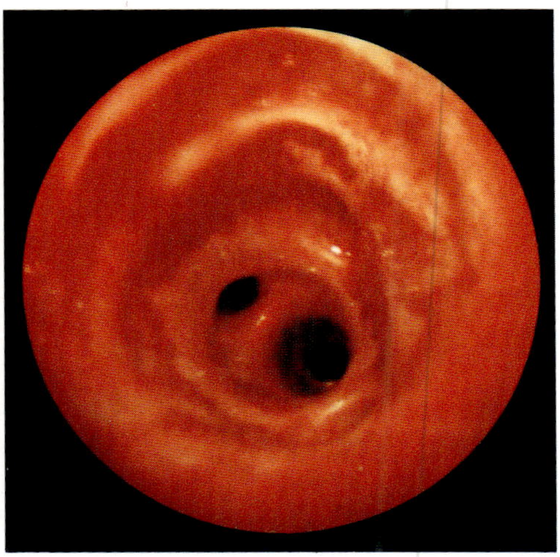

154 Chronic bronchitis with pseudomembranous secretions

155 Carina of a patient with chronic bronchitis, showing the atrophied mucous membrane and enlarged submucosal gland openings

156 Spur of the left upper lobe bronchial orifice. The atrophied mucous membrane discloses the underlying fibrous frame of the bronchus

157 View into the left upper lobe bronchial orifice through the 30°-angled telescope, showing the atrophied mucous membrane in a patient with chronic bronchitis. Note the enlarged openings of the submucosal glands and the petechial hemorrhages marked by the sucker in the superior aspect of this view

158 Distortion of the left lower lobe bronchus produced by severe saccular bronchiectasis of the lower lobe. Note the granulomatous mucous membrane signifying chronic inflammatory change

159 Distortion of the right lower lobe bronchus due to bronchiectasis of the right lower lobe. Note the distorted and inflamed right middle lobe bronchial orifice in the absence of associated bronchiectasis of this lobe

154

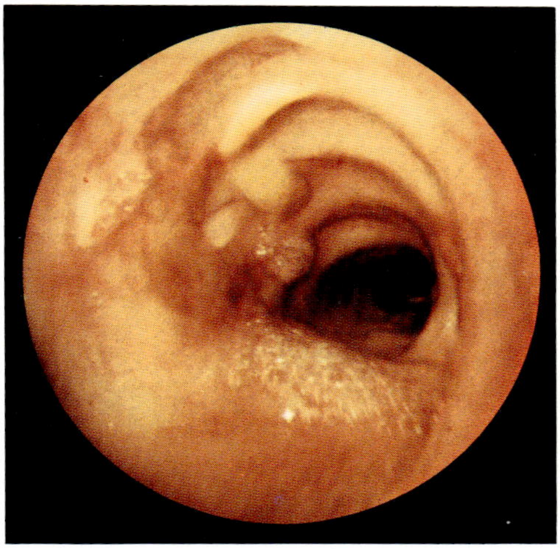

155

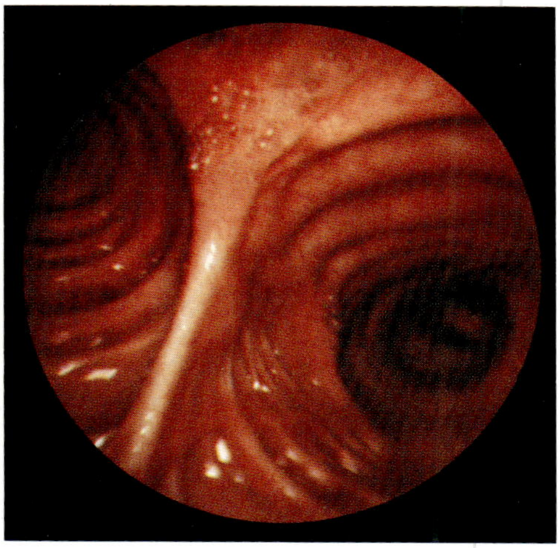

156

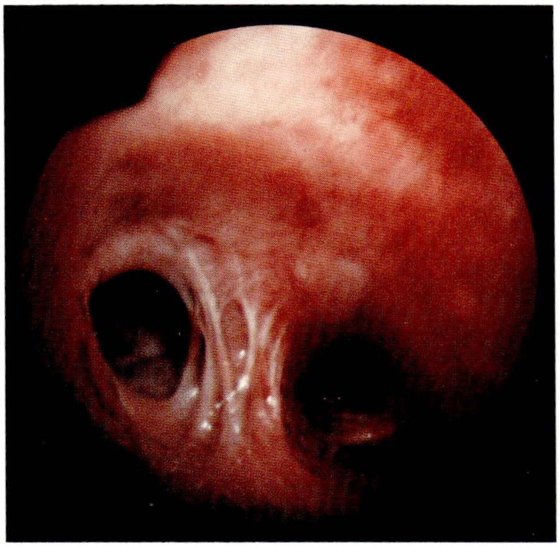

157

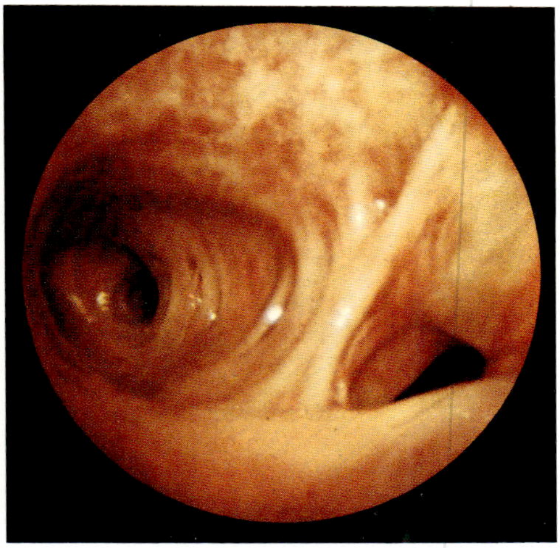

158

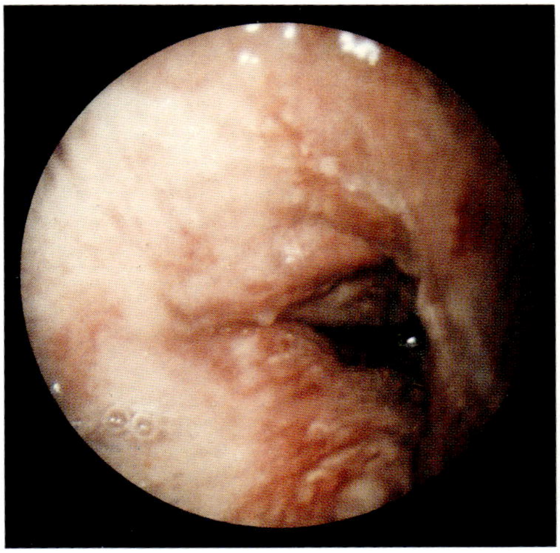

159

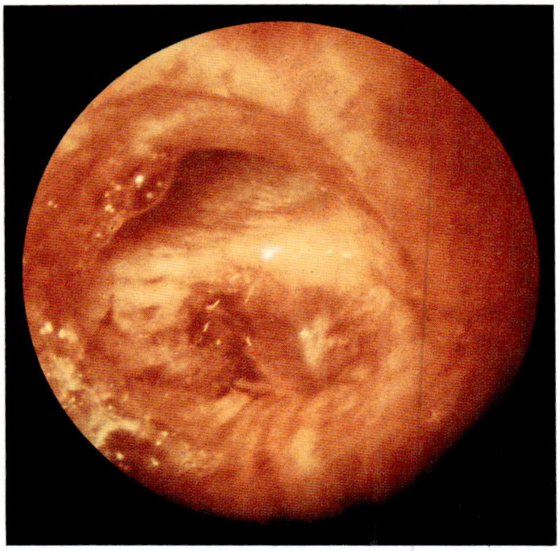

160 Bronchogram of right lung showing filling of all lobar and segmental bronchi

161 Bronchogram of left lung showing filling of all lobar and segmental bronchi

162 Right bronchogram in a child with narrowing of the right intermediate bronchus caused by tuberculous lymph nodes. Note filling of lobar bronchi distally to the narrowed segment

163 Left bronchogram showing an abscess cavity filling from the apical segment of the lower lobe. This is not associated with the tubular bronchiectatic changes demonstrated in the basal bronchi. Note the poor filling of the lingular and upper lobe bronchi

164 The same patient as in Fig. 163, following use of the Sanders air injector to propel contrast media to the periphery, showing complete filling of segmental bronchi

165 Appearances in a child with primary tuberculosis and suspected right middle lobe collapse. On bronchoscopy, the opening to the middle lobe bronchus appeared normal. Bronchography revealed an abnormal but patent middle lobar bronchus

160

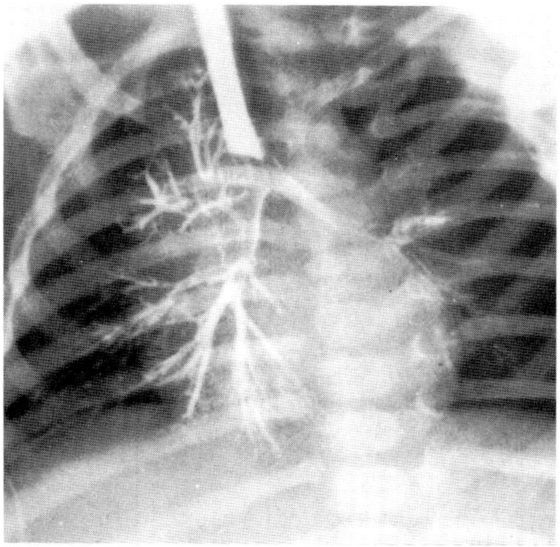

161

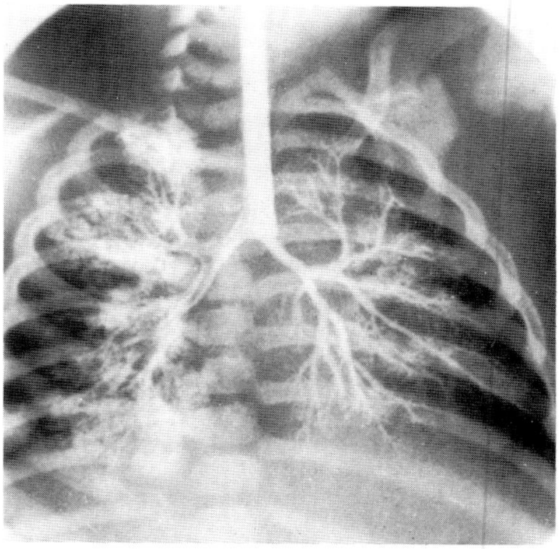

162

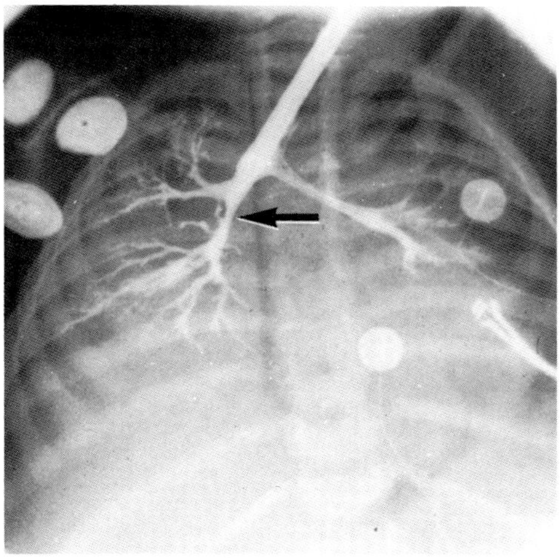

163

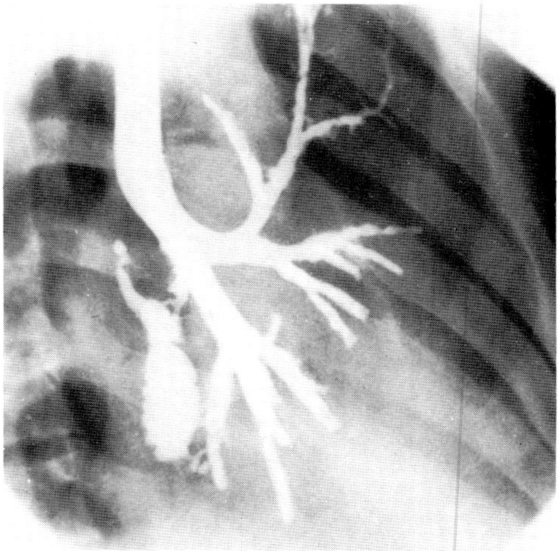

164

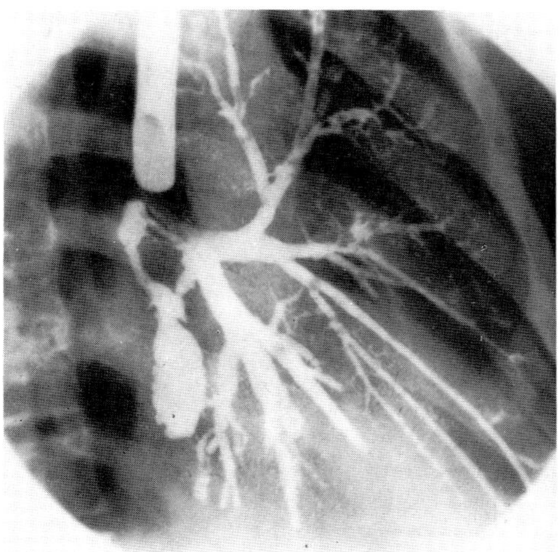

165

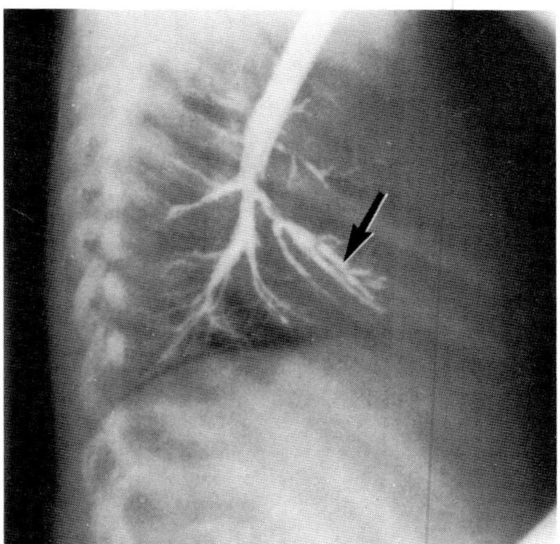

166 Bronchogram in a child who had inhaled sulphuric acid fumes, showing *1* stenosis of the trachea, and *2* stenosis of the left main bronchus

167 Lateral view bronchogram in the same patient as in Fig. 166. The arrow indicates the stenosis of the trachea

168 Selective bronchogram of the right upper lobe employing the Swan-Ganz cardiac catheter

169 Selective bronchogram of the right middle lobe using the Swan-Ganz catheter

170 Selective bronchogram of the lingula of the left lung employing the Swan-Ganz catheter. The arrow points to the inflated balloon at the tip of the catheter

171 Selective bronchogram of the apical segment of the left lower lobe using the Swan-Ganz catheter

166

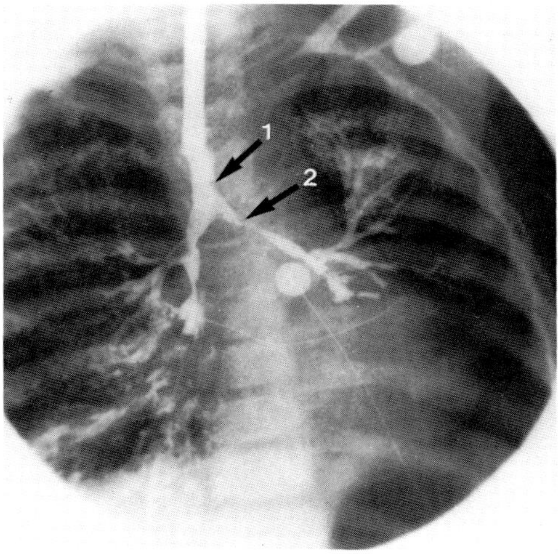


167

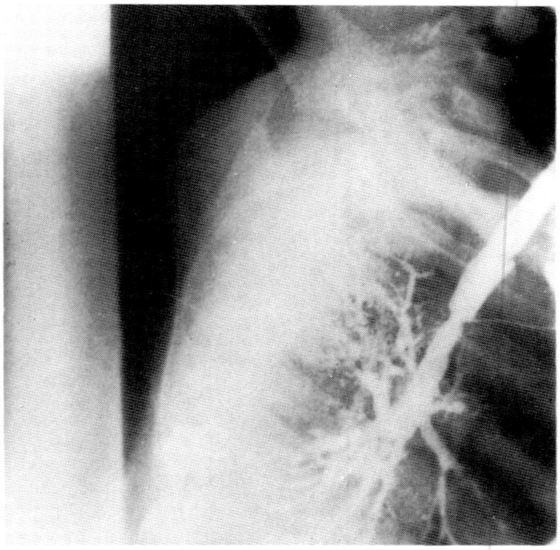

168

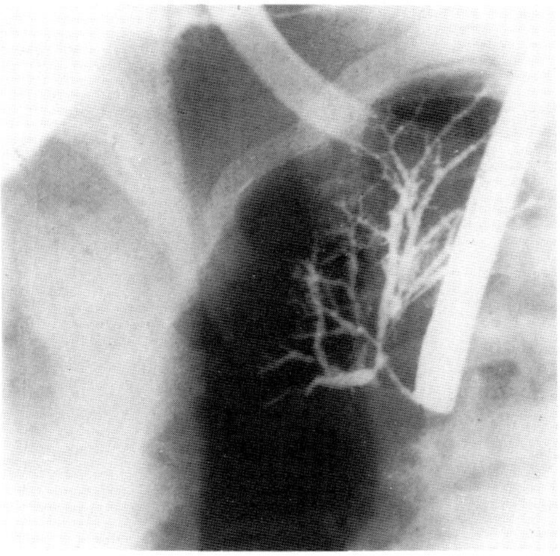

169

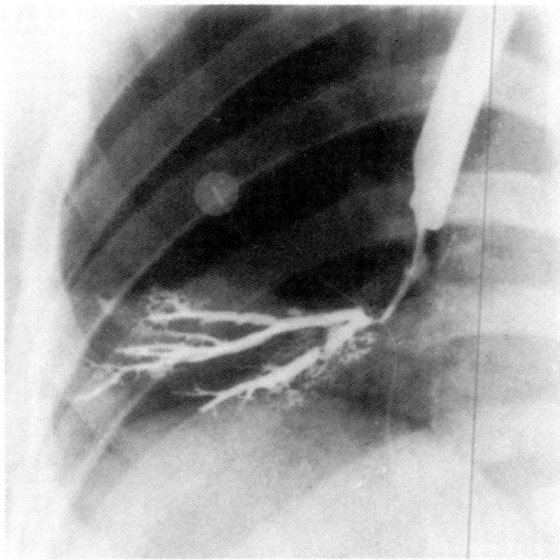

170

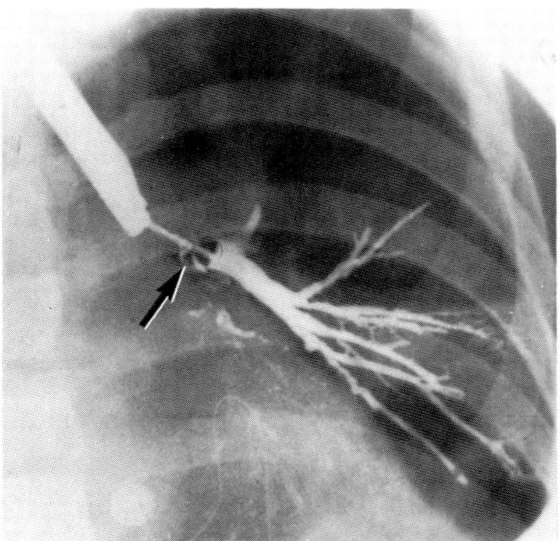

171

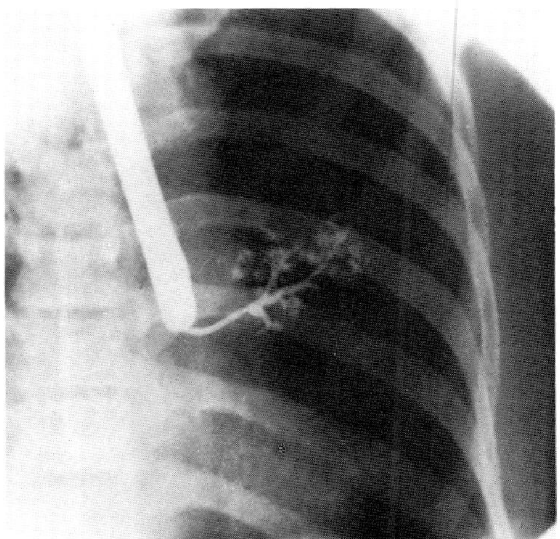

172 Selective bronchogram in a patient with suspected carcinoma of the right middle lobe. The arrow points to a persistent obstruction of a subsegmental bronchus

173 Selective bronchogram of the right upper lobe with nonfilling of the anterior segment

174 Bronchography in the same patient as in Fig. 173, demonstrating how an enlarged infiltrated lymph node *1* exerts pressure on the main right bronchus, the occlusion of the segmental bronchus *2*, and poor filling of the apical segment of the right lower lobe *3* and the right middle lobe *4*

175 The same patient as in Figs. 173 and 174: A bronchogram shows filling of the apical segment of the lower lobe but persistent poor filling of the middle lobar bronchi

176 The same patient as in the preceding three figures: A bronchogram shows normal filling of the right middle lobe following selective catheterization of the lobar bronchus with injection of contrast media

177 Selective bronchogram of left upper lobe showing an area of narrowing and obstruction, where a tumor was seen through the fiberoptic bronchoscope

172

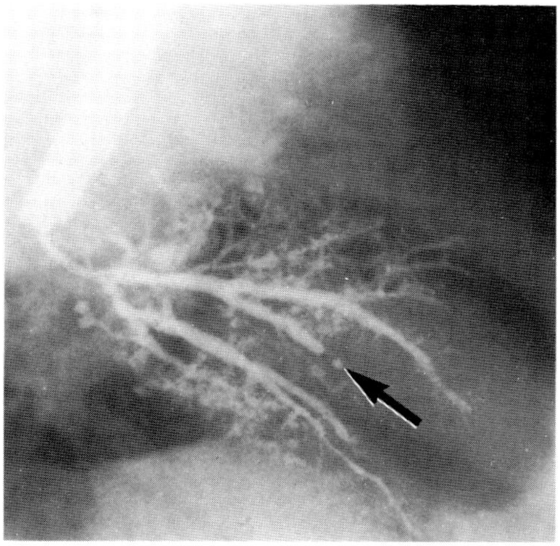

173

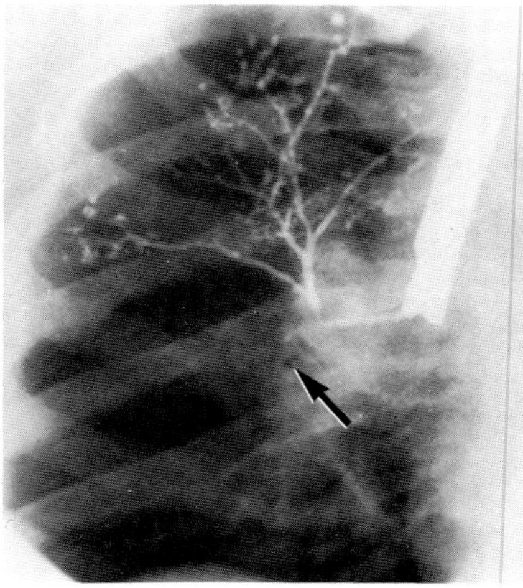

174

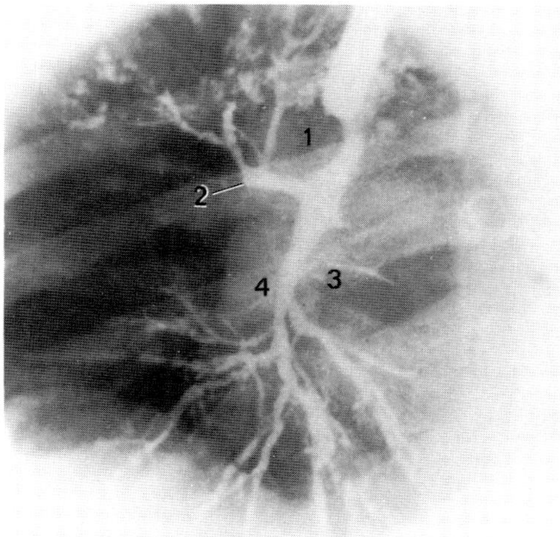


175

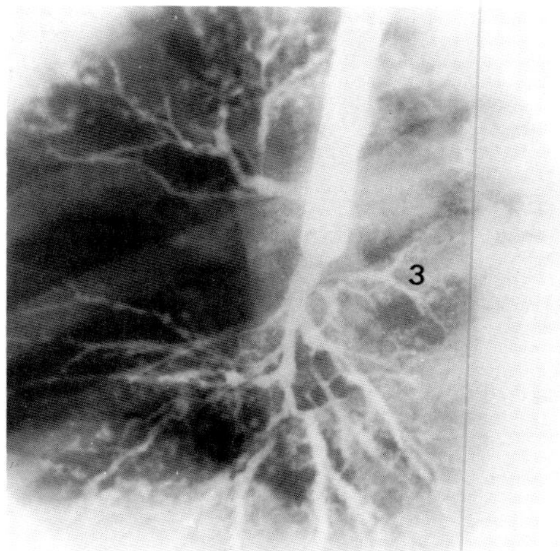


176

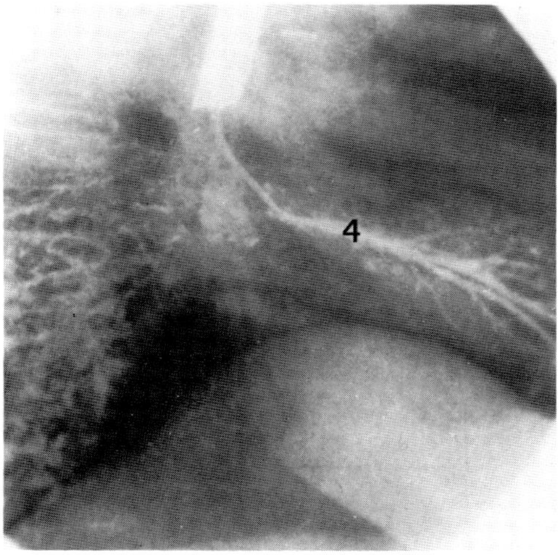


177

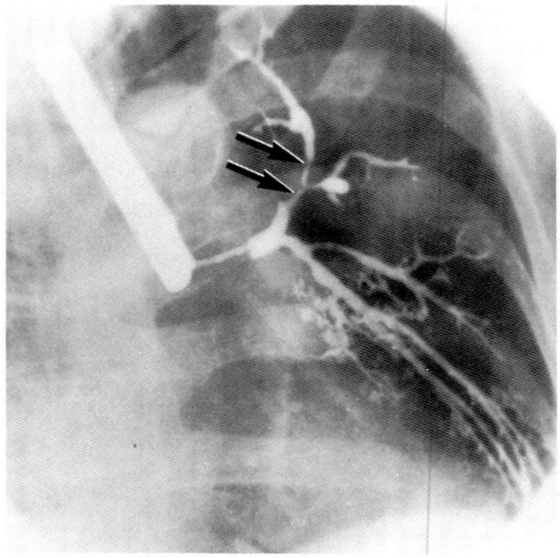

178 Selective bronchogram of the left upper lobe, showing obstruction of the inferior segmental bronchus of the lingula

179 Selective bronchogram of the apical segment of the left upper lobe, to demonstrate, as part of the preoperative assessment of the patient, the size of an abscess cavity and the extent of the associated lung destruction

180 Lateral supine bronchographic view obtained in the same patient as illustrated in Fig. 179. Note the fluid level in the abscess cavity and the presence of a satellite cavity

181 Bronchogram showing saccular bronchiectasis and associated destruction of the left lung. This is an inspiratory view

182 A bronchogram recorded during forced expiration in the same patient as illustrated in Fig. 181 demonstrates functional narrowing down of the bronchiectatic cavities and bronchi, which resulted in effective drainage of the lung (see text)

178

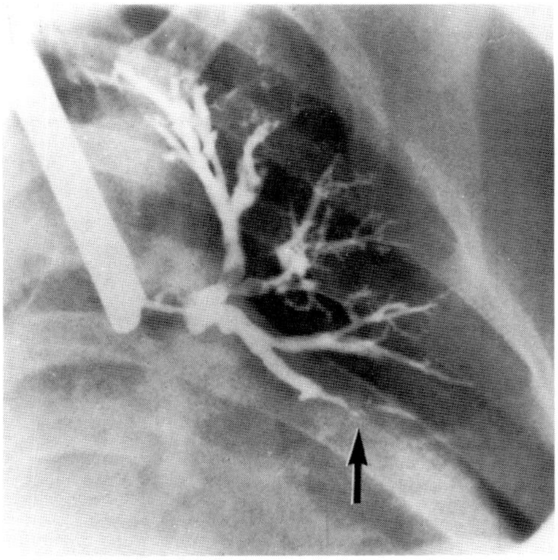

179

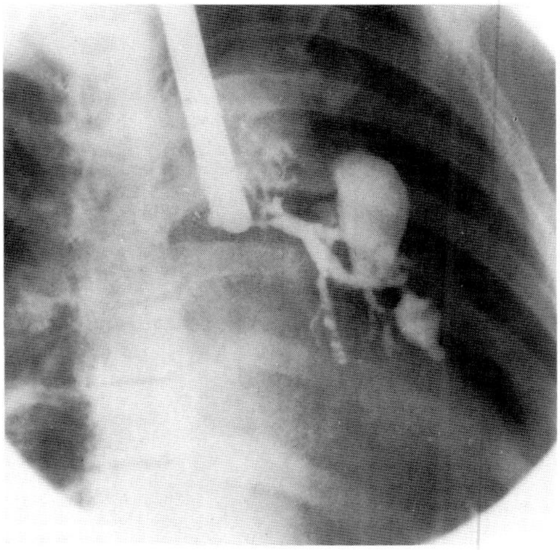

180

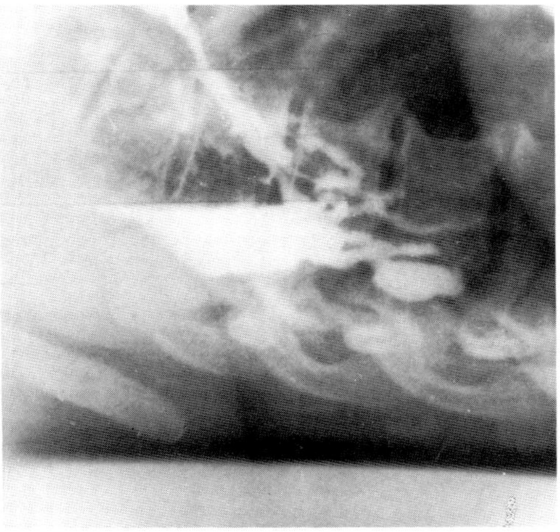

181

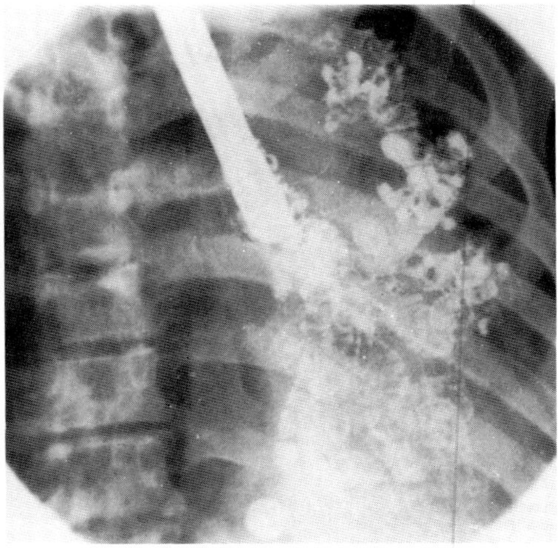

182

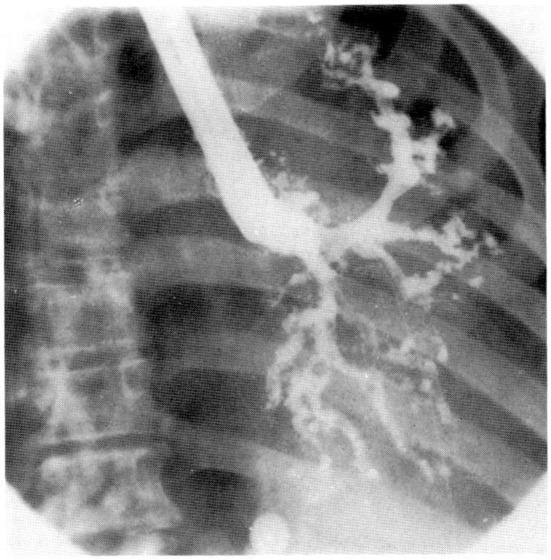

# *Subject Index*

Page numbers in **boldface** refer to illustration pages

# Ergebnisse der Inneren Medizin und Kinderheilkunde

Advances in Internal Medicine and Pediatrics
Neue Folge
Herausgeber: P. Frick, G.-A. von Harnack, G. A. Martini, A. Prader, R. Schoen, H. P. Wolff

*Band 36*

44 Abbildungen, 5 Schemata. IV, 206 Seiten. 1974
ISBN 3-540-06818-X

*Inhaltsübersicht:* A. Junod: The Lung as a Chemical Filter. – A. Hany: Asbestose. – D. Wessinghage, K. Miehlke: Die chronische Polyarthritis. Veränderungen – operative und konservative Behandlung.

# Advances in Cardiopulmonary Resuscitation

The Wolf Creek Conference, 1975

Editor: P. Safar
Associate Editor: J. O. Elam

97 figures, XVI, 302 pages. 1977
ISBN 3-540-90234-1

*Contents:* The Pre-Arrest Period. – Airway Obstruction and Respiratory Arrest. – Circulatory Arrest. – Drugs in Cardiopulmonary Resuscitation. – Electrocardiography, Pacing, Defibrillation. – The Immediate Post-Resuscitative Period. – Special Considerations. – Historic Vignettes.

This book is more than the Proceedings of the Wolf-Creek Conference on Advances in Resuscitation. The 46 papers of this volume have been written by 24 authors, most of whom were first or second generation pioneers of modern resuscitation, which began in the 1950's. The topics include the pre-arrest period, airway obstruction and respiratory arrest; circulatory arrest; drugs in CPR; electrocardiography-pacing-defibrillation, the immediate post-resuscitative period (with special emphasis on recent advances in brain resuscitation); special considerations (such as massive hemorrhage, neardrowning, educational and legal considerations); and historic vignettes. Some of the papers have primarily teaching value; others bring new, as yet unpublished, data, and others are unique because of unpublished historic facts they convery. The historic vignettes and discussions of other papers include stories and quotes of deceased pioneers in resuscitation, such as Claude Beck and William Kouwenhoven. The 24 Clinican Scientists who met for this "think tank" pre-distributed manuscripts in order to take account of the present developments in CPR, and to have a look into the future. Their edited manuscripts and discussions published in this volume represent a synthesis of recent scientific, clinical and educational advances of respiratory, circulatory and cerebral resuscitation.

# Experimental Lung Cancer

Carcinogenesis and Bioassays

International Symposium hold at the Battelle Seattle Research Center, Seattle, WA., USA, June 23–26, 1974
Editors: E. Karbe, J. F. Park

312 figures, 44 tables. XI, 611 pages. 1974
ISBN 3-540-06996-8
Distribution rights for Japan:
Maruzen Co. Ltd. Tokyo

This book contains 58 reports by international scientists on animal experiments relative to inhalation carcinogenesis and models for testing inhaled carcinogens. The main emphasis is on methods of application, syncarcinogenesis, the carcinogenic effects of tobacco smoke and radioactive materials, in-vitro methods, and the histology of experimentally induced tumours in the respiratory organs of various animal species.

# Anaesthesiology and Resuscitation

Anaesthesiologie und Wiederbelebung
Anesthésiologie et Réanimation
Editors: R. Frey, F. Kern, O. Mayrhofer
Managing Editor: H. Bergmann
Volume 105

H. Reineke

# Lungenveränderungen während Dauerbeatmung

26 Abbildungen, 7 Tabellen. VII, 56 Seiten. 1977
ISBN 3-540-08101-1

*Inhaltsübersicht:* Einleitung: Problematik. Fragestellung. – Methodik: Material und Gruppen, Versuchsanordnung. Theoretische Aspekte zur Meßtechnik direkt registrierter Einzelwerte. Meßgeräte. Einzelmeßwerte. Berechnete Größen. Morphologische Untersuchungen. Statistik. – Ergebnisse: Lungenfunktion. Lungenmorphologie. – Diskussion: Methodik. Ergebnisse. – Zusammenfassung. – Summary. – Literatur. – Sachverzeichnis.

Springer-Verlag
Berlin
Heidelberg
New York